TOTEM AND TABOO

Founded by C. K. Ogden

The International Library of Psychology

PSYCHOANALYSIS
In 28 Volumes

TOTEM AND TABOO

Some Points of Agreement Between the Mental Lives of Savages and Neurotics

SIGMUND FREUD

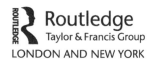

Routledge
Taylor & Francis Group
LONDON AND NEW YORK

First published in 1950
by Routledge
2 Park Square, Milton Park, Abingdon, Oxfordshire OX14 4RN
711 Third Avenue, New York, NY 10017

First issued in paperback 2014

Routledge is an imprint of the Taylor and Francis Group, an informa business

© 1950 Routledge and Kegan Paul, Ltd, Translated by James
Strachey

British Library Cataloguing in Publication Data
A CIP catalogue record for this book
is available from the British Library

Totem and Taboo
ISBN 0415-21090-9
Psychoanalysis: 28 Volumes
ISBN 0415-21132-8
The International Library of Psychology: 204 Volumes
ISBN 0415-19132-7

ISBN 13: 978-1-138-87557-9 (pbk)
ISBN 13: 978-0-415-21090-4 (hbk)

Contents

Translator's Note

AS Freud explains in his own preface, the four essays comprised in this volume were originally published in the pages of the periodical *Imago* (Vienna) under the title 'Über einige Übereinstimmungen im Seelenleben der Wilden und der Neurotiker' ['On Some Points of Agreement between the Mental Lives of Savages and Neurotics']—the first and second essays in Vol. I (1912) and the third and fourth in Vol. II (1913). All four essays were collected and published under the new title of *Totem und Tabu* in 1913 (Vienna, Hugo Heller). New editions appeared in 1920, 1922 and 1934 and the work was included in Volume X of Freud's *Gesammelte Schriften* (Vienna, 1924) and as Volume IX of his *Gesammelte Werke* (London, 1940). None of these later editions show any variations of substance from the original one. An English translation by A. A. Brill was published in New York in 1918 (London, 1919). The book has also been translated into Hungarian (1918), Spanish (1923), Portuguese (*n.d.*), French (1924), Japanese (twice, 1930 and 1934) and Hebrew (1939). The last of these was introduced by a specially written preface, which, on account of its particular interest, I have included in this volume.

For the purposes of the present, entirely new, version I have made an effort to verify all quotations and references so far as possible; and I have put right a considerable number of inaccuracies which had crept into the German editions. Particulars of all works referred to in the text will be found in a list at the end of the volume. The responsibility for any matter printed between square brackets is mine.

My grateful thanks are due to Miss Anna Freud for her critical revision of the entire translation, and to Mr. Roger Money-Kyrle for reading through the typescript and making many helpful suggestions.

J. S.

Preface

THE four essays that follow were originally published (under a heading which serves as the present book's sub-title) in the first two volumes of *Imago*, a periodical issued under my direction. They represent a first attempt on my part at applying the point of view and the findings of psycho-analysis to some unsolved problems of social psychology [*Völkerpsychologie*]. Thus they offer a methodological contrast on the one hand to Wilhelm Wundt's extensive work, which applies the hypotheses and working methods of *non*-analytic psychology to the same purposes, and on the other hand to the writings of the Zurich school of psycho-analysis, which endeavour, on the contrary, to solve the problems of individual psychology with the help of material derived from social psychology. (Cf. Jung, 1912 and 1913.) I readily confess that it was from these two sources that I received the first stimulus for my own essays.

I am fully conscious of the deficiencies of these studies. I need not mention those which are necessarily characteristic of pioneering work; but others require a word of explanation. The four essays collected in these pages aim at arousing the interest of a fairly wide circle of educated readers, but they cannot in fact be understood and appreciated except by those few who are no longer strangers to the essential nature of psycho-analysis. They seek to bridge the gap between students of such subjects as social anthropology, philology and folklore on the one hand, and psycho-analysts on the other. Yet they cannot offer to either side what each lacks—to the former an adequate initiation into the new psychological technique or to the latter a sufficient grasp of the material that awaits treatment. They must therefore rest content with attracting the attention of the two parties and with encouraging a belief that occasional

Preface

co-operation between them could not fail to be of benefit to research.

It will be found that the two principal themes from which the title of this little book is derived—totems and taboos—have not received the same treatment. The analysis of taboos is put forward as an assured and exhaustive attempt at the solution of the problem. The investigation of totemism does no more than declare that 'here is what psycho-analysis can at the moment contribute towards elucidating the problem of the totem'. The difference is related to the fact that taboos still exist among us. Though expressed in a negative form and directed towards another subject-matter, they do not differ in their psychological nature from Kant's 'categorical imperative', which operates in a compulsive fashion and rejects any conscious motives. Totemism, on the contrary, is something alien to our contemporary feelings—a religio-social institution which has been long abandoned as an actuality and replaced by newer forms. It has left only the slightest traces behind it in the religions, manners and customs of the civilized peoples of to-day and has been subject to far-reaching modifications even among the races over which it still holds sway. The social and technical advances in human history have affected taboos far less than the totem.

An attempt is made in this volume to deduce the original meaning of totemism from the vestiges remaining of it in childhood—from the hints of it which emerge in the course of the growth of our own children. The close connection between totems and taboos carries us a step further along the path towards the hypothesis presented in these pages; and if in the end that hypothesis bears a highly improbable appearance, that need be no argument against the possibility of its approximating more or less closely to the reality which it is so hard to reconstruct.

Rome, *September* 1913.

TOTEM AND TABOO

I

The Horror of Incest

PREHISTORIC man, in the various stages of his development, is known to us through the inanimate monuments and implements which he has left behind, through the information about his art, his religion and his attitude towards life which has come to us either directly or by way of tradition handed down in legends, myths and fairy tales, and through the relics of his mode of thought which survive in our own manners and customs. But apart from this, in a certain sense he is still our contemporary. There are men still living who, as we believe, stand very near to primitive man, far nearer than we do, and whom we therefore regard as his direct heirs and representatives. Such is our view of those whom we describe as savages or half-savages; and their mental life must have a peculiar interest for us if we are right in seeing in it a well-preserved picture of an early stage of our own development.

If that supposition is correct, a comparison between the psychology of primitive peoples, as it is taught by social anthropology, and the psychology of neurotics, as it has been revealed by psycho-analysis, will be bound to show numerous points of agreement and will throw new light upon familiar facts in both sciences.

For external as well as for internal reasons, I shall select as the basis of this comparison the tribes which have been described by anthropologists as the most backward and miserable of savages, the aborigines of Australia, the youngest continent, in whose fauna, too, we can still observe much that is archaic and that has perished elsewhere.

The Australian aborigines are regarded as a distinct race, showing neither physical nor linguistic relationship with their nearest neighbours, the Melanesian, Polynesian and Malayan peoples. They do not build houses or permanent shelters; they do not cultivate the soil; they keep no domesticated animals except the dog; they are not even acquainted with the art of making pottery. They live entirely upon the flesh of all kinds of animals which they hunt, and upon roots which they dig. Kings or chiefs are unknown among them; communal affairs are decided by a council of elders. It is highly doubtful whether any religion, in the shape of a worship of higher beings, can be attributed to them. The tribes in the interior of the continent, who have to struggle against the hardest conditions of existence as a result of the scarcity of water, appear to be more primitive in all respects than those living near the coast.

We should certainly not expect that the sexual life of these poor, naked cannibals would be moral in our sense or that their sexual instincts would be subjected to any great degree of restriction. Yet we find that they set before themselves with the most scrupulous care and the most painful severity the aim of avoiding incestuous sexual relations. Indeed, their whole social organization seems to serve that purpose or to have been brought into relation with its attainment.

Among the Australians the place of all the religious and social institutions which they lack is taken by the system of 'totemism'. Australian tribes fall into smaller divisions, or clans, each of which is named after its totem. What is a totem? It is as a rule an animal (whether edible and harmless or dangerous and feared) and more rarely a plant or a natural phenomenon (such as rain or water), which stands in a peculiar relation to the whole clan. In the first place, the totem is the common ancestor of the clan; at the same time it is their guardian spirit and helper, which sends them oracles and, if dangerous to others, recognizes and spares its own children. Conversely, the clansmen are under a sacred obligation (subject to automatic sanctions) not to kill or destroy their totem and to avoid eating its flesh (or deriving benefit from it in other ways). The totemic character is inherent, not in some individual animal or entity, but in all the individuals of a given class. From time to time festivals are celebrated at which the clansmen represent or imitate the motions and attributes of their totem in ceremonial dances.

2

The Horror of Incest

The totem may be inherited either through the female or through the male line. It is possible that originally the former method of descent prevailed everywhere and was only subsequently replaced by the latter. An Australian's relation to his totem is the basis of all his social obligations: it overrides on the one hand his tribal membership and on the other hand his blood relationships.[1]

The totem is not attached to one particular place. The clansmen are distributed in different localities and live peacefully side by side with members of other totem clans.[2]

And now we come at last to the characteristic of the totemic system which has attracted the interest of psycho-analysts. In

[1] 'The Totem bond is stronger than the bond of blood or family in the modern sense.' (Frazer, 1910, 1, 53.)

[2] This highly condensed summary of the totemic system must necessarily be subject to further comments and qualifications. The word 'totem' was first introduced in 1791 (in the form 'totam') from the North American Indians by an Englishman, J. Long. The subject itself has gradually attracted great scientific interest and has produced a copious literature, from which I may select as works of capital importance J. G. Frazer's four-volume *Totemism and Exogamy* (1910) and the writings of Andrew Lang, e.g. *The Secret of the Totem* (1905). The merit of having been the first to recognize the importance of totemism for human prehistory lies with a Scotsman, John Ferguson McLennan (1869–70). Totemic institutions were, or still are, to be observed in operation, not only among the Australians, but also among the North American Indians, among the peoples of Oceania, in the East Indies and in a large part of Africa. It may also be inferred from certain vestigial remains, for which it is otherwise hard to account, that totemism existed at one time among the Aryan and Semitic aboriginal races of Europe and Asia. Many investigators are therefore inclined to regard it as a necessary phase of human development which has been passed through universally.

How did prehistoric men come to adopt totems? How, that is, did they come to make the fact of their being descended from one animal or another the basis of their social obligations and, as we shall see presently, of their sexual restrictions? There are numerous theories on the subject —of which Wundt (1906 [264 ff.]) has given an epitome for German readers—but no agreement. It is my intention to devote a special study before long to the problem of totemism, in which I shall attempt to solve it by the help of a psycho-analytic line of approach. (See the fourth essay in this volume.)

Not only, however, is the *theory* of totemism a matter of dispute; the almost every place where we find totems we also find a law against persons of the same totem having sexual relations with one another and consequently against their marrying.[1] This, then, is 'exogamy', an institution related to totemism.

Strictly enforced as it is, this prohibition is a remarkable one. There is nothing in the concept or attributes of the totem which I have so far mentioned to lead us to anticipate it; so that it is hard to understand how it has become involved in the totemic system. We cannot, therefore, feel surprised that some investigators actually suppose that exogamy had originally—in the earliest times and in its true meaning—nothing to do with totemism, but became attached to it (without there being any underlying connection) at some time when marriage restrictions became necessary. However this may be, the bond between totemism and exogamy exists and is clearly a very firm one.

Some further considerations will make the significance of this prohibition clearer:

(*a*) The violation of the prohibition is not left to what might be called the 'automatic' punishment of the guilty parties, as in the case of other totem prohibitions, such as that against killing the totem animal. It is avenged in the most energetic fashion by the whole clan, as though it were a question of averting some danger that threatened the whole community or some guilt that was pressing upon it. A few sentences from Frazer (1910, **1**, 54) will show how severely such misdeeds are treated by savages who are otherwise far from being moral by our standards:

'In Australia the regular penalty for sexual intercourse with a

facts themselves are scarcely capable of being expressed in genera terms as I have tried to do in the text above. There is scarcely a statement which does not call for exceptions or contradictions. But it must not be forgotten that even the most primitive and conservative races are in some sense *ancient* races and have a long past history behind them during which their original conditions of life have been subject to much development and distortion. So it comes about that in those races in which totemism exists to-day, we may find it in various stages of decay and disintegration or in the process of transition to other social and religious institutions, or again in a stationary condition which may differ greatly from the original one. The difficulty in this last case is to decide whether we should regard the present state of things as a true picture of the significant features of the past or as a secondary distortion of them.

[1] [This sentence is in spaced type in the original.]

person of a forbidden clan is death. It matters not whether the woman be of the same local group or has been captured in war from another tribe; a man of the wrong clan who uses her as his wife is hunted down and killed by his clansmen, and so is the woman; though in some cases, if they succeed in eluding capture for a certain time, the offence may be condoned. In the Ta-ta-thi tribe, New South Wales, in the rare cases which occur, the man is killed but the woman is only beaten or speared, or both, till she is nearly dead; the reason given for not actually killing her being that she was probably coerced. Even in casual amours the clan prohibitions are strictly observed; any violations of these prohibitions "are regarded with the utmost abhorrence and are punished by death".' [Quoted from Cameron (1885, 351.)]

(*b*) Since the same severe punishment is inflicted in the case of passing love-affairs which have not resulted in any children, it seems unlikely that the reasons for the prohibition are of a practical nature.

(*c*) Since totems are hereditary and not changed by marriage, it is easy to follow the consequences of the prohibition. Where, for instance, descent is through the female line, if a man of the Kangaroo totem marries a woman of the Emu totem, all the children, both boys and girls, belong to the Emu clan. The totem regulation will therefore make it impossible for a son of this marriage to have incestuous intercourse with his mother or sisters, who are Emus like himself.[1]

(*d*) But a little more reflection will show that exogamy linked with the totem effects more (and therefore *aims* at more) than the prevention of incest with a man's mother and sisters. It makes sexual intercourse impossible for a man with all the

---

[1] On the other hand, at all events so far as this prohibition is concerned, the father, who is a Kangaroo, is free to commit incest with his daughters, who are Emus. If the totem descended through the *male* line, however, the Kangaroo father would be prohibited from incest with his daughters (since all his children would be Kangaroos), whereas the son would be free to commit incest with his mother. These implications of totem prohibitions suggest that descent through the female line is older than that through the male, since there are grounds for thinking that totem prohibitions were principally directed against the incestuous desires of the son.

B

5

women of his own clan (that is to say with a number of women who are not his blood-relatives) by treating them all as though they *were* his blood-relatives. It is difficult at first sight to see the psychological justification for this very extensive restriction, which goes far beyond anything comparable among civilized peoples. It may be gathered from this, however, that the part played by the totem as common ancestor is taken very seriously. All those who are descended from the same totem are blood-relations. They form a single family, and within that family even the most distant degree of kinship is regarded as an absolute hindrance to sexual intercourse.

We see, then, that these savages have an unusually great horror of incest, or are sensitive on the subject to an unusual degree, and that they combine this with a peculiarity which remains obscure to us—of replacing real blood-relationship by totem kinship. This latter contrast must not, however, be too much exaggerated, and we must remember that the totem prohibitions include that against real incest as a special case.

The riddle of how it came about that the real family was replaced by the totem clan must perhaps remain unsolved till the nature of the totem itself can be explained. At the same time, it is to be observed that if there were a certain degree of freedom of sexual intercourse outside marriage, blood-relationship, and consequently the prevention of incest, would become so uncertain that the prohibition would stand in need of a wider basis. It is therefore worth remarking that Australian customs permit the occurrence, in certain social situations and during certain festivals, of breaches in a man's exclusive conjugal rights over a woman.

Linguistic usage in these Australian tribes[1] exhibits a peculiarity which is no doubt relevant here. For the terms used by them to express the various degrees of kinship do not denote a relation between two individuals but between an individual and a group. This is what L. H. Morgan [1877] named the 'classificatory' system of relationship. Thus a man uses the term 'father' not only for his actual procreator but also for all the other men whom his mother might have married according to tribal law and who therefore might have procreated him; he

[1] As well as in most other totemic communities.

uses the term 'mother' not only for the woman who actually bore him but also for all the other women who might have borne him without transgressing the tribal law; he uses the terms 'brother' and 'sister' not only for the children of his actual parents but also for the children of all those persons who stand in the relation of parents to him in the classificatory sense; and so on. Thus the kinship terms which two Australians apply to each other do not necessarily indicate any consanguinity, as ours would do: they represent social rather than physical relationships. Something approaching the classificatory system is to be found among us when, for instance, children are encouraged to refer to all their parents' friends as 'Uncle' or 'Aunt', or when we speak in a metaphorical sense of 'brothers in Apollo' or 'sisters in Christ'.

Though this use of words strikes us as so puzzling, it is easily explained if we look on it as a survival of the marriage institution which the Rev. L. Fison has called 'group marriage' and which consists in a certain number of men exercising conjugal rights over a certain number of women. The children of such a group marriage would then justly regard one another as brothers and sisters (though they were not all born of the same mother) and would regard all the men in the group as their fathers.

Though some authors, such as Westermarck (1901), have disputed the conclusions which others have drawn from the existence of the classificatory system of relationship, those who have the closest acquaintance with the Australian natives are agreed in regarding that system as a survival from the days of group marriage. Indeed, according to Spencer and Gillen (1899 [64]), a certain form of group marriage exists to this day in the Urabunna and Dieri tribes. Group marriage thus preceded individual marriage among these peoples, and after its disappearance left definite traces behind both in language and customs.

But when once we have put group marriage in the place of individual marriage, the apparently excessive degree of avoidance of incest which we have come across among the same peoples becomes intelligible. Totemic exogamy, the prohibition of sexual intercourse between members of the same clan, appears to have been the appropriate means for preventing group incest; it thus became established and persisted long after its *raison d'être* had ceased.

It may seem that we have thus discovered the motives that led the Australian natives to set up their marriage restrictions; but we have now to learn that the actual state of affairs reveals a far greater, and at first sight a bewildering, complexity. For there are few races in Australia in which the totem barrier is the sole prohibition. Most of them are organized in such a way as to fall into two divisions, known as marriage-classes or 'phratries'. Each of these phratries is exogamous and comprises a number of totem clans. As a rule each phratry is further subdivided into two 'sub-phratries', the whole tribe being thus divided into four, with the sub-phratries intermediate between the phratries and the totem clans.

The following diagram represents the typical organization of an Australian tribe and corresponds to the actual situation in a very large number of cases:

Here the twelve totem clans are divided into four sub-phratries and two phratries. All the divisions are exogamous.[1] Subphratries c and e form an exogamous unit; and so also do subphratries d and f. The result (and therefore the purpose) of these arrangements cannot be doubted: they bring about a still further restriction on the choice of marriage and on sexual liberty. Let us suppose that each clan contains an equal number of members. Then, if only the twelve totem clans existed, each member of a clan would have his choice among $\frac{11}{12}$ of all the women in the tribe. The existence of the two phratries reduces his choice to $\frac{6}{12}$ or $\frac{1}{2}$, for then a man of totem a can only marry a woman of totems 1 to 6. With the introduction of the four subphratries his choice is still further reduced to $\frac{3}{12}$ or $\frac{1}{4}$, for in that

[1] The number of totems is chosen arbitrarily.

case a man of totem *a* is restricted in his choice of a wife to a woman of totems 4, 5 or 6.

The historical relation between the marriage-classes (of which in some tribes there are as many as eight) and the totem clans is completely obscure. It is merely evident that these arrangements are directed towards the same aim as totemic exogamy and pursue it still further. While, however, totemic exogamy gives one the impression of being a sacred ordinance of unknown origin—in short, of being a custom—the complicated institution of the marriage-classes, with their subdivisions and the regulations attaching to them, look more like the result of deliberate legislation, which may perhaps have taken up the task of preventing incest afresh because the influence of the totem was waning. And, while the totemic system is, as we know, the basis of all the other social obligations and moral restrictions of the tribe, the significance of the phratries seems in general not to extend beyond the regulation of marriage choice which is its aim.

The system of marriage-classes in its furthest developments bears witness to an endeavour to go beyond the prevention of natural and group incest and to forbid marriage between still more distant groups of relatives. In this it resembles the Catholic Church, which extended the ancient prohibition against marriage between brothers and sisters to marriage between cousins and even to marriage between those who were merely spiritual relatives [—godfathers, godmothers and godchildren]. (Cf. Lang, 1910–11 [87].)

It would be little to our purpose if we were to follow in detail the extraordinarily involved and obscure discussions on the origin and significance of the marriage-classes and on their relation to the totem. For our purpose it is enough to draw attention to the great care which is devoted by the Australians, as well as by other savage peoples, to the prevention of incest.[1] It must be admitted that these savages are even more sensitive on the subject of incest than we are. They are probably liable to a greater temptation to it and for that reason stand in need of fuller protection.

But the horror of incest shown by these peoples is not satis-

[1] Storfer (1911[16]) has quite recently insisted on this point.

fied by the erection of the institutions which I have described and which seem to be directed principally against group incest. We must add to them a number of 'customs' which regulate the dealings of individuals with their near relatives in our sense of the term, customs which are enforced literally with religious strictness and the purpose of which can scarcely be doubted. These customs or customary prohibitions have been termed 'avoidances'. They extend far beyond the totemic races of Australia; but once again I must ask my readers to be content with a fragmentary extract from the copious material.

In Melanesia restrictive prohibitions of this sort govern a boy's intercourse with his mother and sisters. Thus, for instance, in Lepers' Island, one of the New Hebrides, when a boy has reached a certain age he no longer lives at home, but takes up his quarters in the 'club-house', where he now regularly eats and sleeps. It is true that he may still go to his father's house to ask for food, but if his sister is at home he must go away before eating; if no sister is there he may sit down near the door and eat. If by chance a brother and sister meet in the open, she must run away or hide. If a boy knows that certain footprints in the road are his sister's, he will not follow them, nor will she follow his. Indeed, he will not even utter her name, and will avoid the use of a common word if it forms part of her name. This avoidance begins with the puberty ceremonies and is maintained throughout life. The reserve between a son and his mother increases as the boy grows up and is much more on her side than on his. If his mother brings him food, she does not give it him but puts it down for him to take. In speaking to him she does not *tutoyer* him, but uses the more distant plural forms.[1]

Similar customs prevail in New Caledonia. If a brother and sister happen to meet on a path, the sister will throw herself into the bushes and he will pass on without turning his head.[2]

Among the natives of the Gazelle Peninsula in New Britain a sister, after her marriage, is not allowed to converse with her brother; she never utters his name, but designates him by another word.[3]

[1] Frazer (1910, **2**, 77 f.), quoting Codrington (1891, [232]).
[2] [Frazer (1910, **2**, 78), quoting Lambert (1900, 114).]
[3] Frazer (1910, **2**, 124) [quoting Parkinson (1907, 67 f.)].

The Horror of Incest

In New Mecklenburg cousins of one kind are subject to similar restrictions, as are brothers and sisters. They may not come near each other, may not shake hands and may not give each other presents; but they are allowed to speak to each other at a distance of some paces. The penalty for incest with a sister is death by hanging.[1]

In Fiji these avoidance rules are particularly strict; they affect not only blood sisters but tribal sisters as well. It must strike us as all the more puzzling to hear that these same savages practise sacred orgies, in which precisely these forbidden degrees of kinship seek sexual intercourse—puzzling, that is, unless we prefer to regard the contrast as an explanation of the prohibition.[2]

Among the Battas of Sumatra the rules of avoidance apply to all near relations. 'A Batta, for example, would think it shocking were a brother to escort his sister to an evening party. Even in the presence of others a Batta brother and sister feel embarrassed. If one of them comes into the house, the other will go away. Further, a father may never be alone in the house with his daughter, nor a mother with her son. . . . The Dutch missionary who reports these customs adds that he is sorry to say that from what he knows of the Battas he believes the maintenance of most of these rules to be very necessary.' These people assume as a matter of course that a solitary meeting between a man and a woman will lead to an improper intimacy between them. And since they believe that intercourse between near relations will lead to punishments and calamities of all sorts, they are right to avoid any temptation to trangress these prohibitions.[3]

Curiously enough, among the Barongo of Delagoa Bay, in South Africa, the strictest rules affect a man's relations with his sister-in-law, the wife of his wife's brother. If he meets this formidable person anywhere, he carefully avoids her. He does not eat out of the same dish with her, he speaks to her with embarrassment, does not venture into her hut and greets her in a trembling voice.[4]

---

[1] Frazer (1910, **2**, 130 f.), quoting Peckel (1908 [467]).
[2] Frazer (1910, **2**, 146 ff.), quoting Fison [1885, 27 ff.].
[3] Frazer (1910, **2**, 189) [quoting Joustra (1902, 391 f.)].
[4] Frazer (1910, **2**, 388), quoting [Junod 1898, 73 ff.].

A rule of avoidance with which one would have expected to meet more frequently operates among the A-kamba (or Wakamba) of British East Africa. A girl has to avoid her father between the age of puberty and the time of her marriage. If they meet in the road, she hides while he passes, and she may never go and sit near him. This holds good until the moment of her betrothal. After her marriage she does not avoid her father in any way.[1]

By far the most widespread and strictest avoidance (and the most interesting from the point of view of civilized races) is that which restricts a man's intercourse with his mother-in-law. It is quite general in Australia and also extends over Melanesia, Polynesia and the Negro races of Africa, wherever traces of totemism and the classificatory system of relationship are found and probably still further. In some of these places there are similar prohibitions against a woman having innocent intercourse with her father-in-law; but they are far less usual and severe. In a few isolated cases both parents-in-law are subject to avoidance. Since we are less concerned in the ethnographical extent of this avoidance than in its substance and purpose, I shall once again restrict myself to quoting a few examples.

Among the Melanesians of the Banks' Islands 'these rules of avoidance are very strict and minute. A man will not come near his wife's mother and she will not come near him. If the two chance to meet in a path, the woman will step out of it and stand with her back turned till he has gone by, or perhaps, if it be more convenient, he will move out of the way. At Vanua Lava, in Port Patteson, a man would not even follow his mother-in-law along the beach until the rising tide had washed her footprints from the sand. Yet a man and his mother-in-law may talk to each other at a distance; but a woman will on no account mention the name of her daughter's husband, nor will he name hers.'[2]

In the Solomon Islands, after his marriage a man may neither see nor converse with his mother-in-law. If he meets her, he may not recognize her, but must make off and hide himself as fast as he can.[3]

[1] Frazer (1910, 2, 424) [quoting C. W. Hobley (unpublished MS.)].
[2] Frazer (1910, 2, 76) [quoting Codrington (1891, 42 ff.)].
[3] Frazer (1910, 2, 117), quoting Ribbe (1903 [140 f.]).

The Horror of Incest

Among the Eastern Bantu 'custom requires that a man should "be ashamed of" his wife's mother, that is to say, he must studiously shun her society. He may not enter the same hut with her, and if by chance they meet on a path, one or other turns aside, she perhaps hiding behind a bush, while he screens his face with a shield. If they cannot thus avoid each other, and the mother-in-law has nothing else to cover herself with, she will tie a wisp of grass round her head as a token of ceremonial avoidance. All correspondence between the two has to be carried on either through a third party or by shouting to each other at a distance with some barrier, such as the kraal fence, interposed between them. They may not even pronounce each other's proper name.' (Frazer, 1910, **2**, 385.)

Among the Basoga, a Bantu people who live in the region of the sources of the Nile, a man may only speak to his mother-in-law when she is in another room and out of sight. Incidentally, these people have such a horror of incest that they punish it even when it occurs among their domestic animals. (Frazer, 1910, **2**, 461.)

While there can be no doubt as to the purpose and significance of the other avoidances between near relations, and they are universally regarded as protective measures against incest, the prohibitions affecting a man's intercourse with his mother-in-law have received another interpretation in some quarters. It was with justice regarded as incomprehensible that all these different peoples should feel such great fear of the temptation presented to a man by an elderly woman, who might have been, but in fact was not, his mother. (Crawley, 1902, 405.)

This objection was also raised against the view put forward by Fison [Fison and Howitt, 1880, 104]. He pointed out that certain systems of marriage-classes had gaps in them, as a result of which marriage between a man and his mother-in-law was not theoretically impossible. For that reason, he suggested, a special guarantee against that possibility became necessary.

Sir John Lubbock (1870 [84 f.]) traced back the attitude of a mother-in-law to her son-in-law to the institution of 'marriage by capture'. 'When the capture was a reality', he writes, 'the indignation of the parents would also be real; when it became a mere symbol, the parental anger would be symbolized also, and

13

would be continued even after its origin was forgotten.' Crawley [1902, 406] has no difficulty in showing how insufficiently this attempted explanation covers the details of the observed facts.

Tylor [1889, 246 f.] believes that the treatment given to a son-in-law by his mother-in-law is merely a form of 'cutting' or non-recognition by the wife's family: the man is regarded as an 'outsider' until the first child is born. In the first place, however, the prohibition is not always brought to an end when this occurs. But, apart from this, it may be objected that this explanation throws no light on the fact that the prohibition centres particularly on the *mother*-in-law—that is to say, that it overlooks the factor of sex. Moreover, it takes no account of the attitude of religious horror expressed in the prohibition. (Crawley, 1902, 407.)

A Zulu woman, questioned as to the basis of the prohibition, gave the sensitive reply: 'It is not right that he should see the breasts which suckled his wife.'[1]

As we know, the relation between son-in-law and mother-in-law is also one of the delicate points of family organization in *civilized* communities. That relation is no longer subject to rules of avoidance in the social system of the white peoples of Europe and America; but many disputes and much unpleasantness could often be eliminated if the avoidance still existed as a custom and did not have to be re-erected by individuals. It may be regarded by some Europeans as an act of high wisdom on the part of these savage races that by their rules of avoidance they entirely precluded any contact between two persons brought into this close relationship to each other. There is scarcely room for doubt that something in the psychological relation of a mother-in-law to a son-in-law breeds hostility between them and makes it hard for them to live together. But the fact that in civilized societies mothers-in-law are such a favourite subject for jokes seems to me to suggest that the emotional relation involved includes sharply contrasted components. I believe, that is, that this relation is in fact an 'ambivalent' one, composed of conflicting affectionate and hostile impulses.

Some of those impulses are obvious enough. On the side of the mother-in-law there is reluctance to give up the possession

[1] Crawley (1902, 401), quoting Leslie (1875 [141]).

of her daughter, distrust of the stranger to whom she is to be handed over, an impulse to retain the dominating position which she has occupied in her own house. On the man's side there is a determination not to submit any longer to someone else's will, jealousy of anyone who possessed his wife's affection before he did, and, last but not least, an unwillingness to allow anything to interfere with the illusory over-valuation bred of his sexual feelings. The figure of his mother-in-law usually causes such an interference, for she has many features which remind him of her daughter and yet lacks all the charms of youth, beauty and spiritual freshness which endear his wife to him.

But we are able to bring forward other motives than these, thanks to the knowledge of concealed mental impulses which we have acquired from the psycho-analytic examination of individual human beings. A woman whose psycho-sexual needs should find satisfaction in her marriage and her family life is often threatened with the danger of being left unsatisfied, because her marriage relation has come to a premature end and because of the uneventfulness of her emotional life. A mother, as she grows older, saves herself from this by putting herself in her children's place, by identifying herself with them; and this she does by making their emotional experiences her own. Parents are said to stay young with their children, and that is indeed one of the most precious psychological gains that parents derive from their children. Where a marriage is childless, the wife has lost one of the things which might be of most help to her in tolerating the resignation that her own marriage demands from her. A mother's sympathetic identification with her daughter can easily go so far that she herself falls in love with the man her daughter loves; and in glaring instances this may lead to severe forms of neurotic illness as a result of her violent mental struggles against this emotional situation. In any case, it very frequently happens that a mother-in-law is subject to an *impulse* to fall in love in this way, and this impulse itself or an opposing trend are added to the tumult of conflicting forces in her mind. And very often the unkind, sadistic components of her love are directed on to her son-in-law in order that the forbidden, affectionate ones may be the more severely suppressed.

A man's relation to his mother-in-law is complicated by similar impulses, though they have another source. It is regularly found that he chose his mother as the object of his love, and perhaps his sister as well, before passing on to his final choice. Because of the barrier that exists against incest, his love is deflected from the two figures on whom his affection was centred in his childhood on to an outside object that is modelled upon them. The place of his own and his sister's mother is taken by his mother-in-law. He has an impulse to fall back upon his original choice, though everything in him fights against it. His horror of incest insists that the genealogical history of his choice of an object for his love shall not be recalled. His repudiation of this impulse is also facilitated by the fact that his mother-in-law is only a contemporary figure; he has not known her all his life, so that there is no unchangeable picture of her preserved in his unconscious. A streak of irritability and malevolence that is apt to be present in the medley of his feelings leads us to suspect that she does in fact offer him a temptation to incest; and this is confirmed by the not uncommon event of a man openly falling in love with the woman who is later to be his mother-in-law before transferring his love to her daughter.

I can see nothing against the presumption that it is precisely this incestuous factor in the relation that provides savages with the motive for their rules of avoidance between son-in-law and mother-in-law. Thus the explanation which we should adopt for these strictly enforced avoidances among primitive peoples is that put forward by Fison [see p. 13], which regards them merely as a further protection against possible incest. The same explanation holds good of all other avoidances, between both blood and tribal relations. The only difference would be that in the case of blood relations the possibility of incest is an immediate one and the intention to prevent it may be conscious; in the other cases, including that of a man's relation to his mother-in-law, the possibility of incest would seem to be a temptation in phantasy set in motion through the agency of unconscious connecting links.

There has been little opportunity in the preceding pages for showing how new light can be thrown upon the facts of social psychology by the adoption of a psycho-analytic method of approach: for the horror of incest displayed by savages has long been recognized as such and stands in need of no further interpretation. All that I have been able to add to our understanding of it is to emphasize the fact that it is essentially an *infantile* feature and that it reveals a striking agreement with the mental life of neurotic patients. Psycho-analysis has taught us that a boy's earliest choice of objects for his love is incestuous and that those objects are forbidden ones—his mother and his sister. We have learnt, too, the manner in which, as he grows up, he liberates himself from this incestuous attraction. A neurotic, on the other hand, invariably exhibits some degree of psychical infantilism. He has either failed to get free from the psycho-sexual conditions that prevailed in his childhood or he has returned to them—two possibilities which may be summed up as developmental inhibition and regression. Thus incestuous fixations of libido continue to play (or begin once more to play) the principal part in his unconscious mental life. We have arrived at the point of regarding a child's relation to his parents, dominated as it is by incestuous longings, as the nuclear complex of neurosis. This revelation of the importance of incest in neurosis is naturally received with universal scepticism by adults and normal people. Similar expressions of disbelief, for instance, inevitably greet the writings of Otto Rank [e.g. 1907 and 1912], which have brought more and more evidence to show the extent to which the interest of creative writers centres round the theme of incest and how the same theme, in countless variations and distortions, provides the subject-matter of poetry. We are driven to believe that this rejection is principally a product of the distaste which human beings feel for their early incestuous wishes, now overtaken by repression. It is therefore of no small importance that we are able to show that these same incestuous wishes, which are later destined to become unconscious, are still regarded by savage peoples as immediate perils against which the most severe measures of defence must be enforced.

II

Taboo and
Emotional Ambivalence

(1)

'TABOO' is a Polynesian word. It is difficult for us to find a translation for it, since the concept connoted by it is one which we no longer possess. It was still current among the ancient Romans, whose '*sacer*' was the same as the Polynesian 'taboo'. So, too, the '*ἄγος*' of the Greeks and the '*kadesh*' of the Hebrews must have had the same meaning as is expressed in 'taboo' by the Polynesians and in analogous terms by many other races in America, Africa (Madagascar) and North and Central Asia.

The meaning of 'taboo', as we see it, diverges in two contrary directions. To us it means, on the one hand, 'sacred', 'consecrated', and on the other 'uncanny', 'dangerous', 'forbidden', 'unclean'. The converse of 'taboo' in Polynesian is '*noa*', which means 'common' or 'generally accessible'. Thus 'taboo' has about it a sense of something unapproachable, and it is principally expressed in prohibitions and restrictions. Our collocation 'holy dread' would often coincide in meaning with 'taboo'.

Taboo restrictions are distinct from religious or moral prohibitions. They are not based upon any divine ordinance, but may be said to impose themselves on their own account. They differ from moral prohibitions in that they fall into no system that declares quite generally that certain abstinences must be observed and gives reasons for that necessity. Taboo prohibitions have no grounds and are of unknown origin. Though they are unintelligible to *us*, to those who are dominated by them they are taken as a matter of course.

Wundt (1906, 308) describes taboo as the oldest human unwritten code of laws. It is generally supposed that taboo is older

18

than gods and dates back to a period before any kind of religion existed.

Since we need an impartial account of taboo to submit to psycho-analytic examination, I shall now give some extracts and summaries of portions of the article 'Taboo' in the *Encyclopaedia Britannica* (1910–11),[1] the author of which was Northcote W. Thomas, the anthropologist.

'Properly speaking taboo includes only (*a*) the sacred (or unclean) character of person or things, (*b*) the kind of prohibition which results from this character, and (*c*) the sanctity (or uncleanness) which results from a violation of the prohibition. The converse of taboo in Polynesia is *noa* and allied forms, which mean "general" or "common". . . .

'Various classes of taboo in the wider sense may be distinguished: (i) natural or direct, the result of *mana* (mysterious power) inherent in a person or thing; (ii) communicated or indirect, equally the result of *mana*, but (*a*) acquired or (*b*) imposed by a priest, chief or other person; (iii) intermediate, where both factors are present, as in the appropriation of a wife to her husband. . . .' The term is also applied to other ritual restrictions, but what is better described as a 'religious interdiction' should not be referred to as taboo.

'The objects of taboo are many: (i) direct taboos aim at (*a*) the protection of important persons—chiefs, priests, etc.—and things against harm; (*b*) the safeguarding of the weak—women, children and common people generally—from the powerful *mana* (magical influence) of chiefs and priests; (*c*) the provision against the dangers incurred by handling or coming in contact with corpses, by eating certain foods, etc.; (*d*) the guarding the chief acts of life—birth, initiation, marriage and sexual functions, etc., against interference; (*e*) the securing of human beings against the wrath or power of gods and spirits;[2] (*f*) the securing of unborn infants and young children, who stand in a specially sympathetic relation with one or both parents, from the consequences of certain actions, and more especially from

---

[1] This includes a bibliography of the chief literature on the subject.

[2] In the present context this use of the term 'taboo' may be disregarded as not being a primary one.

the communication of qualities supposed to be derived from certain foods. (ii) Taboos are imposed in order to secure against thieves the property of an individual, his fields, tools, etc. . . .'

The punishment for the violation of a taboo was no doubt originally left to an internal, automatic agency: the violated taboo itself took vengeance. When, at a later stage, ideas of gods and spirits arose, with whom taboo became associated, the penalty was expected to follow automatically from the divine power. In other cases, probably as a result of a further evolution of the concept, society itself took over the punishment of offenders, whose conduct had brought their fellows into danger. Thus the earliest human penal systems may be traced back to taboo.

'The violation of a taboo makes the offender himself taboo. . . .' Certain of the dangers brought into existence by the violation may be averted by acts of atonement and purification.

The source of taboo is attributed to a peculiar magical power which is inherent in persons and spirits and can be conveyed by them through the medium of inanimate objects. 'Persons or things which are regarded as taboo may be compared to objects charged with electricity; they are the seat of a tremendous power which is transmissible by contact, and may be liberated with destructive effect if the organisms which provoke its discharge are too weak to resist it; the result of a violation of a taboo depends partly on the strength of the magical influence inherent in the taboo object or person, partly on the strength of the opposing *mana* of the violator of the taboo. Thus, kings and chiefs are possessed of great power, and it is death for their subjects to address them directly; but a minister or other person of greater *mana* than common can approach them unharmed, and can in turn be approached by their inferiors without risk. . . . So too indirect taboos depend for their strength on the *mana* of him who imposes them; if it is a chief or a priest, they are more powerful than those imposed by a common person. . . .'

It is no doubt the transmissibility of taboo which accounts for the attempts to throw it off by suitable purificatory ceremonies.

Taboos may be permanent or temporary. Among the former are those attaching to priests and chiefs, as well as to dead persons and anything belonging to them. Temporary taboos may be attached to certain particular states, such as menstruation and child-birth, to warriors before and after an expedition, or to special activities such as fishing and hunting. A general taboo may (like a Papal Interdict) be imposed upon a whole region and may then last for many years.

If I judge my readers' feelings aright, I think it is safe to say that in spite of all that they have now heard about taboo they still have very little idea of the meaning of the term or of what place to give it in their thoughts. This is no doubt due to the insufficiency of the information I have given them and to my having omitted to discuss the relation between taboo and superstition, the belief in spirits, and religion. On the other hand, I am afraid a more detailed account of what is known about taboo would have been even more confusing, and I can assure them that in fact the whole subject is highly obscure.

What we are concerned with, then, is a number of prohibitions to which these primitive races are subjected. Every sort of thing is forbidden; but they have no idea why, and it does not occur to them to raise the question. On the contrary, they submit to the prohibitions as though they were a matter of course and feel convinced that any violation of them will be automatically met by the direst punishment. We have trustworthy stories of how any unwitting violation of one of these prohibitions is in fact automatically punished. An innocent wrong-doer, who may, for instance, have eaten a forbidden animal, falls into a deep depression, anticipates death and then dies in bitter earnest. These prohibitions are mainly directed against liberty of enjoyment and against freedom of movement and communication. In some cases they have an intelligible meaning and are clearly aimed at abstinences and renunciations. But in other cases their subject-matter is quite incomprehensible; they are concerned with trivial details and seem to be of a purely ceremonial nature.

Behind all these prohibitions there seems to be something in the nature of a theory that they are necessary because certain persons and things are charged with a dangerous power, which can be transferred through contact with them, almost like an infection. The *quantity* of this dangerous attribute also plays a part.

C

Some people or things have more of it than others and the danger is actually proportional to the difference of potential of the charges. The strangest fact seems to be that anyone who has transgressed one of these prohibitions himself acquires the characteristic of being prohibited—as though the whole of the dangerous charge had been transferred over to him. This power is attached to all *special* individuals, such as kings, priests or newborn babies, to all *exceptional* states, such as the physical states of menstruation, puberty or birth, and to all *uncanny* things, such as sickness and death and what is associated with them through their power of infection or contagion.

The word 'taboo' denotes everything, whether a person or a place or a thing or a transitory condition, which is the vehicle or source of this mysterious attribute. It also denotes the prohibitions arising from the same attribute. And, finally, it has a connotation which includes alike 'sacred' and 'above the ordinary', as well as 'dangerous', 'unclean' and 'uncanny'.

This word and the system denoted by it give expression to a group of mental attitudes and ideas which seem remote indeed from our understanding. In particular, there would seem to be no possibility of our coming into closer contact with them without examining the belief in ghosts and spirits which is characteristic of these low levels of culture.

Why, it may be asked at this point, should we concern ourselves at all with this riddle of taboo? Not only, I think, because it is worth while trying to solve *any* psychological problem for its own sake, but for other reasons as well. It may begin to dawn on us that the taboos of the savage Polynesians are after all not so remote from us as we were inclined to think at first, that the moral and conventional prohibitions by which we ourselves are governed may have some essential relationship with these primitive taboos and that an explanation of taboo might throw a light upon the obscure origin of our own 'categorical imperative'.

Accordingly, we shall be particularly interested to hear the views of so notable an investigator as Wilhelm Wundt on the subject of taboo, especially as he promises 'to trace back the concept of taboo to its earliest roots' (1906, 301).

Taboo and Emotional Ambivalence

Wundt writes of that concept that 'it comprises all of the usages in which is expressed a dread of certain objects related to cult ideas or of actions connected with them'. (Ibid., 237.) And, in another passage: 'If we understand by it [taboo], in accordance with the general meaning of the word, every prohibition (whether laid down in usage or custom or in explicitly formulated laws) against touching an object or making use of it for one's own purposes or against using certain proscribed words . . .' then, he goes on, there can be no race and no level of culture which has escaped the ill-effects of taboo. [Ibid., 301.]

Wundt next proceeds to explain why it seems to him advisable to study the nature of taboo in the primitive conditions of the Australian savages rather than in the higher culture of the Polynesian peoples. [Ibid., 302.] He divides the taboo prohibitions among the Australians into three classes, according as they affect animals, human beings or other objects. The taboos on animals, which consist essentially of prohibitions against killing and eating them, constitute the nucleus of *Totemism*. [Ibid., 303.][1] The second class of taboos, those directed towards human beings, are of an entirely different kind. They are restricted in the first instance to circumstances in which the person on whom the taboo is imposed finds himself in an unusual situation. Thus young men are taboo at their initiation ceremonies, women are taboo during menstruation and immediately after giving birth; so too new-born babies, sick persons and, above all, the dead are taboo. A man's property which is in his constant use is permanently taboo to all other men: his clothing, for instance, his tools and weapons. Included in a man's most personal property, in Australia, is the new name which he received when he was a boy at his initiation. It is taboo and must be kept secret. The third class of taboos, which are imposed on trees, plants, houses and localities, are less stable. They appear to follow a rule that anything that is uncanny or provokes dread for any reason becomes subject to taboo. [Ibid., 304.]

The modifications shown by taboo in the richer culture of Polynesia and the Malay Archipelago are, as Wundt himself is obliged to admit, not very profound. The more marked social

[1] Cf. the first and fourth essays in this volume.

23

differences among these peoples find expression in the fact that chiefs, kings and priests exercise a specially effective taboo and are themselves subject to a taboo of the greatest force. [Ibid., 305–6.]

But, adds Wundt, the true sources of taboo lie deeper than in the interests of the privileged classes: 'they have their origin in the source of the most primitive and at the same time most lasting of human instincts—in fear of "demonic" powers.' (Ibid., 307.) 'Taboo is originally nothing other than the objectified fear of the "demonic" power which is believed to lie hidden in a tabooed object. The taboo prohibits anything that may provoke that power and commands that, if it has been injured, whether wittingly or unwittingly, the demon's vengeance must be averted.' [Ibid., 308.]

Little by little, we are told, taboo then grows into a force with a basis of its own, independent of the belief in demons. It develops into the rule of custom and tradition and finally of law. 'But the unspoken command underlying all the prohibitions of taboo, with their numberless variations according to the time and place, is originally one and one only: "Beware of the wrath of demons!" ' [Loc. cit.]

Wundt informs us, then, that taboo is an expression and derivative of the belief of primitive peoples in 'demonic' power. Later, he tells us, it freed itself from this root and remained a power simply because it *was* a power—from a kind of mental conservatism. And thereafter it itself became the root of our moral precepts and of our laws. Though the first of these assertions may provoke little contradiction, I believe I shall be expressing the thoughts of many readers when I say that Wundt's explanation comes as something of a disappointment. This is surely not tracing back the concept of taboo to its sources or revealing its earliest roots. Neither fear nor demons can be regarded by psychology as 'earliest' things, impervious to any attempt at discovering their antecedents. It would be another matter if demons really existed. But we know that, like gods, they are creations of the human mind: they were made by something and out of something.

Wundt has important views on the double significance of taboo, though these are not very clearly expressed. According to him, the distinction between 'sacred' and 'unclean' did not exist in the primitive beginnings of taboo. For that very reason those concepts were at that stage without the peculiar significance which they could only acquire when they became opposed to each other. Animals, human beings or localities on which a taboo was imposed were 'demonic', not 'sacred', nor, therefore, in the sense which was later acquired, 'unclean'. It is precisely this neutral and intermediate meaning—'demonic' or 'what may not be touched'—that is appropriately expressed by the word 'taboo', since it stresses a characteristic which remains common for all time both to what is sacred and to what is unclean: the dread of contact with it. The persistence, however, of this important common characteristic is at the same time evidence that the ground covered by the two was originally one and that it was only as a result of further influences that it became differentiated and eventually developed into opposites. [Ibid., 309.]

According to Wundt, this original characteristic of taboo—the belief in a 'demonic' power which lies hidden in an object and which, if the object is touched or used unlawfully, takes its vengeance by casting a spell over the wrong-doer—is still wholly and solely 'objectified fear'. That fear has not yet split up into the two forms into which it later develops: veneration and horror. [Ibid., 310.]

But how did this split take place? Through the transplanting, so Wundt tells us, of the taboo ordinances from the sphere of demons into the sphere of belief in gods. [Ibid., 311.] The contrast between 'sacred' and 'unclean' coincides with a succession of two stages of mythology. The earlier of these stages did not completely disappear when the second one was reached but persisted in what was regarded as an inferior and eventually a contemptible form. [Ibid., 312.] It is, he says, a general law of mythology that a stage which has been passed, for the very reason that it has been overcome and driven under by a superior stage, persists in an inferior form alongside the later one, so that the objects of its veneration turn into objects of horror. [Ibid., 313.]

The remainder of Wundt's discussion deals with the relation of the concept of taboo to purification and sacrifice.

Totem and Taboo

(2)

Anyone approaching the problem of taboo from the angle of psycho-analysis, that is to say, of the investigation of the unconscious portion of the individual mind, will recognize, after a moment's reflection, that these phenomena are far from unfamiliar to him. He has come across people who have created for themselves individual taboo prohibitions of this very kind and who obey them just as strictly as savages obey the communal taboos of their tribe or society. If he were not already accustomed to describing such people as 'obsessional' patients, he would find 'taboo sickness' a most appropriate name for their condition. Having learnt so much, however, about this obsessional sickness from psycho-analytic examination—its clinical ætiology and the essence of its psychical mechanism—he can scarcely refrain from applying the knowledge he has thus acquired to the parallel sociological phenomenon.

A warning must be uttered at this point. The similarity between taboo and obsessional sickness may be no more than a matter of externals; it may apply only to the *forms* in which they are manifested and not extend to their essential character. Nature delights in making use of the same forms in the most various biological connections: as it does, for instance, in the appearance of branch-like structures both in coral and in plants, and indeed in some forms of crystal and in certain chemical precipitates. It would obviously be hasty and unprofitable to infer the existence of any internal relationship from such points of agreement as these, which merely derive from the operation of the same mechanical causes. We shall bear this warning in mind, but we need not be deterred by it from proceeding with our comparison.

The most obvious and striking point of agreement between the obsessional prohibitions of neurotics and taboos is that these prohibitions are equally lacking in motive and equally puzzling in their origin. Having made their appearance at some unspecified moment, they are forcibly maintained by an irresistible fear. No external threat of punishment is required, for there is an internal certainty, a moral conviction, that any violation will

26

lead to intolerable disaster. The most that an obsessional patient can say on this point is that he has an undefined feeling that some particular person in his environment will be injured as a result of the violation. Nothing is known of the nature of the injury; and indeed even this wretchedly small amount of information is more often obtained in connection with the expiatory and defensive actions which we shall have to discuss later than with the prohibitions themselves.

As in the case of taboo, the principal prohibition, the nucleus of the neurosis, is against touching; and thence it is sometimes known as 'touching phobia' or '*délire du toucher*'. The prohibition does not merely apply to immediate physical contact but has an extent as wide as the metaphorical use of the phrase 'to come in contact with'. Anything that directs the patient's thoughts to the forbidden object, anything that brings him into intellectual contact with it, is just as much prohibited as direct physical contact. This same extension also occurs in the case of taboo.

The purpose of some of the prohibitions is immediately obvious. Others, on the contrary, strike us as incomprehensible, senseless and silly, and prohibitions of this latter sort are described as 'ceremonial'. This distinction, too, is found in the observances of taboo. [See p. 21.]

Obsessional prohibitions are extremely liable to displacement. They extend from one object to another along whatever paths the context may provide, and this new object then becomes, to use the apt expression of one of my women patients, 'impossible'—till at last the whole world lies under an embargo of 'impossibility'. Obsessional patients behave as though the 'impossible' persons and things were carriers of a dangerous infection liable to be spread by contact on to everything in their neighbourhood. I have already [p. 21] drawn attention to the same characteristic capacity for contagion and transference in my description of taboo. We know, too, that anyone who violates a taboo by coming into contact with something that is taboo becomes taboo himself and that then no one may come into contact with *him*.

I will now put side by side two instances of the transference (or, as it is better to say, the *displacement*) of a prohibition. One of these is taken from the life of the Maoris and the other from an observation of my own on a female obsessional patient. 'A Maori chief would not blow a fire with his mouth; for his sacred breath would communicate its sanctity to the fire, which would pass it on to the pot on the fire, which would pass it on to the meat in the pot, which would pass it on to the man who ate the meat, which was in the pot, which stood on the fire, which was breathed on by the chief; so that the eater, infected by the chief's breath conveyed through these intermediaries, would surely die.'[1]

My patient's husband purchased a household article of some kind and brought it home with him. She insisted that it should be removed or it would make the room she lived in 'impossible'. For she had heard that the article had been bought in a shop situated in, let us say, 'Smith' Street.[2] 'Smith', however, was the married name of a woman friend of hers who lived in a distant town and whom she had known in her youth under her maiden name. This friend of hers was at the moment 'impossible' or taboo. Consequently the article that had been purchased here in Vienna was as taboo as the friend herself with whom she must not come into contact.

Obsessional prohibitions involve just as extensive renunciations and restrictions in the lives of those who are subject to them as do taboo prohibitions; but some of them can be lifted if certain actions are performed. Thereafter, these actions *must* be performed: they become compulsive or obsessive acts, and there can be no doubt that they are in the nature of expiation, penance, defensive measures and purification. The commonest of these obsessive acts is washing in water ('washing mania'). Some taboo prohibitions can be replaced in just the same way; or rather their violation can be made good by a similar 'ceremonial'; and here again lustration with water is the preferred method.

Let us now summarize the points in which agreement between taboo usages and obsessional symptoms is most clearly shown: (1) the fact that the prohibitions lack any assignable motive; (2) the fact that they are maintained by an internal necessity; (3) the fact that they are easily displaceable and that there is a risk of infection from the prohibited object; and (4) the fact that they

---

[1] Frazer (1911*b*, 136) [quoting Taylor (1870, 165)].
[2] ['*Hirschengasse*' and '*Hirsch*' in the original.]

give rise to injunctions for the performance of ceremonial acts.

Now both the clinical history and the psychical mechanism of obsessional neurosis have become known to us through psychoanalysis. The clinical history of a typical case of 'touching phobia' is as follows. Quite at the beginning, in very early childhood, the patient shows a strong *desire* to touch, the aim of which is of a far more specialized kind that one would have been inclined to expect. This desire is promptly met by an *external* prohibition against carrying out that particular kind of touching.[1] The prohibition is accepted, since it finds support from powerful *internal* forces,[2] and proves stronger than the instinct which is seeking to express itself in the touching. In consequence, however, of the child's primitive psychical constitution, the prohibition does not succeed in *abolishing* the instinct. Its only result is to *repress* the instinct (the desire to touch) and banish it into the unconscious. Both the prohibition and the instinct persist: the instinct because it has only been repressed and not abolished, and the prohibition because, if it ceased, the instinct would force its way through into consciousness and into actual operation. A situation is created which remains undealt with—a psychical fixation—and everything else follows from the continuing conflict between the prohibition and the instinct.

The principal characteristic of the psychological constellation which becomes fixed in this way is what might be described as the subject's *ambivalent*[3] attitude towards a single object, or rather towards one act in connection with that object. He is constantly wishing to perform this act (the touching), [and looks on it as his supreme enjoyment, but he must not perform it] and detests it as well.[4] The conflict between these two currents cannot be promptly settled because—there is no other way of putting it—they are localized in the subject's mind in such a manner that they cannot come up against each other. The pro-

[1] Both the desire and the prohibition relate to the child's touching his own genitals.

[2] That is, from the child's loving relation to the authors of the prohibition.

[3] To borrow the apt term coined by Bleuler.

[4] [From the Second Edition (1920) onwards, the words in square brackets were, perhaps accidentally, omitted.]

hibition is noisily conscious, while the persistent desire to touch is unconscious and the subject knows nothing of it. If it were not for this psychological factor, an ambivalence like this could neither last so long nor lead to such consequences.

In our clinical history of a case we have insisted that the imposition of the prohibition in very early childhood is the determining point; a similar importance attaches in the subsequent developments to the mechanism of repression at the same early age. As a result of the repression which has been enforced and which involves a loss of memory—an amnesia—the motives for the prohibition (which is conscious) remain unknown; and all attempts at disposing of it by intellectual processess must fail, since they cannot find any base of attack. The prohibition owes its strength and its obsessive character precisely to its unconscious opponent, the concealed and undiminished desire—that is to say, to an internal necessity inaccessible to conscious inspection. The ease with which the prohibition can be transferred and extended reflects a process which falls in with the unconscious desire and is greatly facilitated by the psychological conditions that prevail in the unconscious. The instinctual desire is constantly shifting in order to escape from the *impasse* and endeavours to find substitutes—substitute objects and substitute acts—in place of the prohibited ones. In consequence of this, the prohibition itself shifts about as well, and extends to any new aims which the forbidden impulse may adopt. Any fresh advance made by the repressed libido is answered by a fresh sharpening of the prohibition. The mutual inhibition of the two conflicting forces produces a need for discharge, for reducing the prevailing tension; and to this may be attributed the reason for the performance of obsessive acts. In the case of a neurosis these are clearly compromise actions: from one point of view they are evidences of remorse, efforts at expiation, and so on, while on the other hand they are at the same time substitutive acts to compensate the instinct for what has been prohibited. It is a law of neurotic illness that these obsessive acts fall more and more under the sway of the instinct and approach nearer and nearer to the activity which was originally prohibited.

Let us now make the experiment of treating taboo as though

Taboo and Emotional Ambivalence

it were of the same nature as an obsessional prohibition in one
of our patients. We must make it clear beforehand, however,
that many of the taboo prohibitions that come under our notice
are of a secondary, displaced and distorted kind, and that we
shall have to be satisfied if we can throw only a little light on the
most fundamental and significant taboos. Moreover, the differences between the situation of a savage and of a neurotic are no
doubt of sufficient importance to make any exact agreement impossible and to prevent our carrying the comparison to the
point of identity in every detail.

In the first place, then, it must be said that there is no sense in
asking savages to tell us the real reason for their prohibitions—
the origin of taboo. It follows from our postulates that they cannot answer, since their real reason must be 'unconscious'. We
can, however, reconstruct the history of taboo as follows on the
model of obsessional prohibitions. Taboos, we must suppose, are
prohibitions of primæval antiquity which were at some time
externally imposed upon a generation of primitive men; they
must, that is to say, no doubt have been impressed on them
violently by the previous generation. These prohibitions must
have concerned activities towards which there was a strong inclination. They must then have persisted from generation to
generation, perhaps merely as a result of tradition transmitted
through parental and social authority. Possibly, however, in
later generations they may have become 'organized' as an inherited psychical endowment. Who can decide whether such
things as 'innate ideas' exist, or whether in the present instance
they have operated, either alone or in conjunction with educa-
tion, to bring about the permanent fixing of taboos? But one
thing would certainly follow from the persistence of the taboo,
namely that the original desire to do the prohibited thing must
also still persist among the tribes concerned. They must therefore have an ambivalent attitude towards their taboos. In their
unconscious there is nothing they would like more than to violate them, but they are afraid to do so; they are afraid precisely
because they would like to, and the fear is stronger than the
desire. The desire is unconscious, however, in every individual
member of the tribe just as it is in neurotics.

The most ancient and important taboo prohibitions are the

31

two basic laws of totemism: not to kill the totem animal and to avoid sexual intercourse with members of the totem clan of the opposite sex.

These, then, must be the oldest and most powerful of human desires. We cannot hope to understand this or test our hypothesis on these two examples, so long as we are totally ignorant of the meaning and origin of the totemic system. But the wording of these two taboos and the fact of their concurrence will remind anyone acquainted with the findings of psycho-analytic investigations on individuals of something quite definite, which psycho-analysts regard as the centre-point of childhood wishes and as the nucleus of neuroses.[1]

The multiplicity of the manifestations of taboo, which have led to the attempts at classification that I have already mentioned, are reduced to a single unity by our thesis: the basis of taboo is a prohibited action, for performing which a strong inclination exists in the unconscious.

We have heard [see p. 22], though without understanding it, that anyone who does what is forbidden, that is, who violates a taboo, becomes taboo himself. How is this to be brought into line with the fact that taboo attaches not only to a person who has done what is forbidden but also to persons in particular states, to the states themselves, as well as to impersonal objects? What can the dangerous attribute be which remains the same under all these different conditions? There is only one thing it can be: the quality of exciting men's ambivalence and *tempting* them to transgress the prohibition.

Anyone who has violated a taboo becomes taboo himself because he possesses the dangerous quality of tempting others to follow his example: why should *he* be allowed to do what is forbidden to others? Thus he is truly contagious in that every example encourages imitation, and for that reason he himself must be shunned.

But a person who has not violated any taboo may yet be permanently or temporarily taboo because he is in a state which possesses the quality of arousing forbidden desires in others and of awakening a conflict of ambivalence in them. The majority of

[1] Cf. my forthcoming study upon totemism, to which I have referred more than once in these pages (the fourth essay in this volume).

exceptional positions and exceptional states [see p. 22] are of this kind and possess this dangerous power. The king or chief arouses envy on account of his privileges: everyone, perhaps, would like to be a king. Dead men, new-born babies and women menstruating or in labour stimulate desires by their special helplessness; a man who has just reached maturity stimulates them by the promise of new enjoyment. For that reason all of these persons and all of these states are taboo, since temptation must be resisted.

Now, too, we can understand why the amounts of *mana* possessed by different persons can be subtracted from one another and can to some extent cancel one another out [see p. 20]. A king's taboo is too strong for one of his subjects because the social difference between them is too great. But a minister may without any harm serve as an intermediary between them. If we translate this from the language of taboo into that of normal psychology, it means something like this. A subject, who dreads the great temptation presented to him by contact with the king, can perhaps tolerate dealings with an official whom he does not need to envy so much and whose position may even seem attainable to him. A minister, again, can mitigate his envy of the king by reflecting on the power which he himself wields. So it comes about that smaller differences between the amounts of the tempting magical force possessed by two people are less to be feared than greater ones.

It is equally clear why it is that the violation of certain taboo prohibitions constitutes a social danger which must be punished or atoned for by *all* the members of the community if they are not all to suffer injury [see p. 20]. If we replace the unconscious desires by conscious impulses we shall see that the danger is a real one. It lies in the risk of imitation, which would quickly lead to the dissolution of the community. If the violation were not avenged by the other members they would become aware that they wanted to act in the same way as the transgressor.

We cannot be surprised at the fact that, in the restrictions of taboo, touching plays a part similar to the one which it plays in 'touching phobias', though the secret meaning of the prohibition cannot be of such a specialized nature in taboo as it is in the neurosis. Touching is the first step towards obtaining any sort of control over, or attempting to make use of, a person or object.

We have translated the contagious power inherent in taboo into the possession of some attribute likely to produce temptation or encourage imitation. This does not appear to tally with the fact that the contagious character of taboo is shown chiefly by its transmissibility on to material objects, which then themselves become carriers of taboo.

This transmissibility of taboo is a reflection of the tendency, on which we have already remarked, for the unconscious instinct in the neurosis to shift constantly along associative paths on to new objects. Our attention is thus directed to the fact that the dangerous magical force of *mana* corresponds to two powers of a more realistic sort: the power of reminding a man of his own prohibited wishes and the apparently more important one of inducing him to transgress the prohibition in obedience to those wishes. These two functions can be reduced to one, however, if we suppose that in a primitive mind the awakening of the memory of a forbidden action is naturally linked with the awakening of an impulse to put that action into effect. Thus recollection and temptation come together again. It must be admitted, too, that, in so far as the example of a man transgressing a prohibition tempts another man to do the same, disobedience to prohibitions spreads like a contagion, in just the same way as a taboo is transferred from a person to a material object and from one material object to another.

If the violation of a taboo can be made good by atonement or expiation, which involve the renunciation of some possession or some freedom, this proves that obedience to the taboo injunction meant in itself the renunciation of something desirable. Emancipation from one renunciation is made up for by the imposition of another one elsewhere. This leads us to conclude that atonement is a more fundamental factor than purification in the ceremonials of taboo.

I will now sum up the respects in which light has been thrown on the nature of taboo by comparing it with the obsessional prohibitions of neurotics. Taboo is a primæval prohibition forcibly imposed (by some authority) from outside, and directed against the most powerful longings to which human beings are subject. The desire to violate it persists in their unconscious; those who obey the taboo have an ambivalent attitude to what the taboo prohibits. The magical power that is attributed to taboo is based on the capacity for arousing temptation; and it acts like a contagion because examples are contagious and because the prohibited desire in the unconscious shifts from one thing to another. The fact that the violation of a taboo can be atoned for by a renunciation shows that renunciation lies at the basis of obedience to taboo.

(3)

What we now want to discover is how much value is to be attributed to the parallel we have drawn between taboo and obsessional neurosis and to the view of taboo which we have based on that parallel. Their value must clearly depend on whether the view we have put forward has any advantages over others, and whether it gives us a clearer understanding of taboo than we could otherwise reach. We may be inclined to feel that we have given sufficient evidence of the applicability of our view in what has already been said; yet we must attempt to strengthen the evidence by entering into our explanation of taboo prohibitions and usages in greater detail.

There is also another path open to us. We can start an inquiry as to whether some of the hypotheses which we have carried over from neuroses to taboo or some of the results to which that procedure has led us may not be directly verifiable in the phenomena of taboo. But we must decide what we are to look for. Our assertion that taboo originated in a primæval prohibition imposed at one time or other by some external authority is obviously incapable of demonstration. What we shall rather endeavour to confirm, therefore, are the psychological determinants of taboo, which we have learnt to know from obsessional neurosis. How did we arrive at our knowledge of these psychological factors in the case of the neurosis? Through the analytical study of its symptoms, and particularly of obsessional acts, defensive measures and obsessional commands. We found that they showed every sign of being derived from *ambivalent* im-

35

pulses, either corresponding simultaneously to *both* a wish and a counter-wish or operating predominantly on behalf of *one* of the two opposing trends. If, now, we could succeed in demonstrating that ambivalence, that is, the ascendancy of opposing trends, is also to be found in the observances of taboo, or if we could point to some of them which, like obsessional acts, give simultaneous expression to both currents, we should have established the psychological agreement between taboo and obsessional neurosis in what is perhaps their most important feature.

The two fundamental prohibitions of taboo are, as I have already remarked, inaccessible to our analysis owing to their connection with totemism; while certain others of its injunctions are of a secondary nature and consequently useless for our purpose. For taboo has become the ordinary method of legislation in the communities affected by it and it has come to serve social purposes which are certainly more recent than taboo itself: such, for instance, are the taboos imposed by chiefs and priests for the protection of their own property and privileges. There nevertheless remain a large group of observances on which our investigation can be made. From these I shall select the taboos attaching (*a*) to enemies, (*b*) to chiefs and (*c*) to the dead; and I shall take the material for our examination from the excellent collection included by Frazer in *Taboo and the Perils of the Soul* (1911*b*), the second part of his great work *The Golden Bough*.

(*a*) *The Treatment of Enemies*

We may be inclined to suppose that savage and half-savage races are guilty of uninhibited and ruthless cruelty towards their enemies. We shall be greatly interested to learn, then, that even in their case the killing of a man is governed by a number of observances which are included among the usages of taboo. These observances fall easily into four groups. They demand (1) the appeasement of the slain enemy, (2) restrictions upon the slayer, (3) acts of expiation and purification by him and (4) certain ceremonial observances. Our incomplete information on the subject does not enable us to determine with certainty how general or the reverse these usages may be among the peoples concerned; but for our purposes this is a matter of indifference. It may safely be assumed, in any case, that what we have before us are not isolated peculiarities but widespread usages.

The rites of *appeasement* performed in the island of Timor, when a warlike expedition has returned in triumph bringing the heads of the vanquished foe, are particularly remarkable, since in addition to them the leader of the expedition is submitted to severe restrictions (see below, p. 39). On the occasion of the expedition's return, sacrifices are offered to appease the souls of the men whose heads have been taken. 'The people think that some misfortune would befall the victor were such offerings omitted. Moreover, a part of the ceremony consists of a dance accompanied by a song, in which the death of the slain man is lamented and his forgiveness is entreated. "Be not angry", they say, "because your head is here with us; had we been less lucky, our heads might now have been exposed in your village. We have offered the sacrifice to appease you. Your spirit may now rest and leave us in peace. Why were you our enemy? Would it not have been better that we should remain friends? Then your blood would not have been spilt and your head would not have been cut off." '[1] The same is true of the people of Paloo, in Celebes. So, too, 'the Gallas [of East Africa] returning from war sacrifice to the jinn or guardian spirits of their slain foes before they will re-enter their own houses'.[2]

Other peoples have found a means for changing their former enemies after their death into guardians, friends and benefactors. This method lies in treating their severed heads with affection, as some of the savage races of Borneo boast of doing. When the Sea Dyaks of Sarawak bring home a head from a successful head-hunting expedition, for months after its arrival it is treated with the greatest consideration and addressed with all the names of endearment of which their language is capable. The most dainty morsels of food are thrust into its mouth, delicacies of all kinds and even cigars. The head is repeatedly implored to hate its former friends and to love its new hosts since it has now become one of them. It would be a great mistake to

[1] Frazer (1911*b*, 166) [quoting Gramberg (1872, 216)].

[2] Frazer (loc. cit.), quoting Paulitschke (1893–6 [**2**, 50, 136]).

suppose that these observances, which strike us as so horrible, are performed with any intention of ridicule.[1]

In several of the savage tribes of North America observers have been struck by the mourning over enemies who have been killed and scalped. When a Choctaw had killed an enemy, he went into mourning for a month during which he was subjected to severe restrictions; and the Dacotas had similar practices. When the Osages, reports a witness, have mourned over their own dead, 'they will mourn for the foe just as if he was a friend'.[2]

Before considering the remaining classes of taboo usages in connection with enemies, we must deal with an obvious objection. It will be argued against us, with Frazer and others, that the grounds for such rites of appeasement are simple enough and have nothing to do with any such thing as 'ambivalence'. These peoples are dominated by a superstitious fear of the ghosts of the slain—a fear which was not unknown in classical antiquity and which was put upon the stage by the great English dramatist in the hallucinations of Macbeth and Richard III. All the rites of appeasement follow logically from this superstition, as well as the restrictions and acts of expiation which will be discussed presently. This view is also supported by the fourth group of these observances, which can only be explained as attempts at driving away the ghosts of the victims that are pursuing their murderers.[3] In addition to this, the savages openly admit their fear of the ghosts of dead enemies and themselves attribute to it the taboo usages which we are discussing.

This objection is indeed an obvious one, and if it covered the whole ground we could save ourselves the trouble of any further attempt at an explanation. I shall put off dealing with it until later, and for the moment I will merely state the alternative view which is derived from the hypothesis based upon our earlier discussions of taboo. The conclusion that we must draw

[1] Frazer (1914, **1**, 295), quoting Low (1848 [206]).
[2] Frazer (1911*b*, 181), quoting Dorsey (1884 [126]).
[3] Frazer (1911*b*, 169–74). These ceremonies consist of beating on shields, shouting and screaming, making noises with musical instruments, etc.

from all these observances is that the impulses which they express towards an enemy are not solely hostile ones. They are also manifestations of remorse, of admiration for the enemy, and of a bad conscience for having killed him. It is difficult to resist the notion that, long before a table of laws was handed down by any god, these savages were in possession of a living commandment: 'Thou shalt not kill', a violation of which would not go unpunished.

Let us now return to the other three groups of taboo observances. *Restrictions* placed upon a victorious slayer are unusually frequent and as a rule severe. In Timor (cf. the rites of appeasement described above, on p. 37) the leader of the expedition is forbidden 'to return at once to his own house. A special hut is prepared for him, in which he has to reside for two months, undergoing bodily and spiritual purification. During this time he may not go to his wife nor feed himself; the food must be put into his mouth by another person.'[1] In some Dyak tribes men returning from a successful expedition are obliged to keep to themselves for several days and abstain from various kinds of food; they may not touch iron nor have any intercourse with women. In Logea, an island in the neighbourhood of New Guinea, 'men who have killed or assisted in killing enemies shut themselves up for about a week in their houses. They must avoid all intercourse with their wives and friends, and they may not touch food with their hands. They may eat vegetable food only, which is brought to them cooked in special pots. The intention of these restrictions is to guard the men against the smell of the blood of the slain; for it is believed that if they smelt the blood they would fall ill and die. In the Toaripi or Motumotu tribe of south-eastern New Guinea a man who has killed another may not go near his wife, and may not touch food with his fingers. He is fed by others, and only with certain kinds of food. These observances last till the new moon.' (Frazer, 1911*b*, 167.)

I shall not attempt to give a complete catalogue of the instances quoted by Frazer of restrictions imposed upon victorious manslayers. I will only remark upon a few more such cases in

[1] Frazer (1911*b*, 166), quoting Müller (1857 [**2**, 252]).

39

which their taboo character is particularly marked or in which the restrictions are accompanied by expiation, purification and other ceremonials.

'Among the Monumbos of German New Guinea anyone who has slain a foe in war becomes thereby "unclean" '—the same term being applied to women who are menstruating or in child-bed. He 'must remain a long time in the men's club-house, while the villagers gather round him and celebrate his victory with dance and song. He may touch nobody, not even his own wife and children; if he were to touch them it is believed that they would be covered with sores. He becomes clean again by washing and using other modes of purification.' [Ibid., 169.]

'Among the Natchez of North America young braves who had taken their first scalps were obliged to observe certain rules of abstinence for six months. They might not sleep with their wives nor eat flesh; their only food was fish and hasty-pudding. . . . When a Choctaw had killed an enemy and taken his scalp, he went into mourning for a month, during which he might not comb his hair, and if his head itched he might not scratch it except with a little stick which he wore fastened to his wrist for the purpose.' [Ibid., 181.]

'When a Pima Indian had killed an Apache, he had to go through severe ceremonies of purification and atonement. During a sixteen-day fast he might not touch meat nor salt, nor look on a blazing fire, nor speak to a human being. He lived alone in the woods, waited on by an old woman, who brought him his scanty dole of food. He bathed often in the river and (as a sign of mourning) kept his head covered with a plaster of mud. On the seventeenth day there was a public ceremony of solemn purification of the man and his weapons. Since the Pima Indians took the taboo on killing much more seriously than their enemies and did not, like them, postpone the expiation and purification till the end of the expedition, their warlike efficiency suffered greatly from their moral strictness, or piety, if that term is preferred. Despite their extreme courage, the Americans found them unsatisfactory allies in their operations against the Apaches.' [Ibid., 182–4.]

However much the details and variations of the ceremonies of expiation and purification after the slaying of enemies might be of interest for deeper research into the subject, I shall break off at this point, since for our present purpose they have nothing more to tell us. I may perhaps suggest that the temporary or permanent isolation of professional executioners, which has persisted to the present day, may belong in this connection. The position of the public hangman in mediæval society offers a good picture of the workings of taboo among savages.[1]

In the accepted explanation of all these observances of appeasement, restriction, expiation and purification, two principles are combined: the extension of the taboo from the slain man on to everything that has come in contact with him and the fear of the slain man's ghost. How these two factors áre to be combined with each other to explain the ceremonials, whether they are to be regarded as of equal weight, whether one is primary and the other secondary, and if so which—none of these questions receives an answer, and indeed it would be hard to find one. We, on the other hand, can lay stress on the *unity* of our view, which derives all of these observances from emotional ambivalence towards the enemy.

(b) *The Taboo upon Rulers*

The attitude of primitive peoples to their chiefs, kings and priests is governed by two basic principles which seem to be complementary rather than contradictory. A ruler 'must not only be guarded, he must also be guarded against'. (Frazer, 1911b, 132.) Both of these ends are secured by innumerable taboo observances. We know already why it is that rulers must be guarded against. It is because they are vehicles of the mysterious and dangerous magical power which is transmitted by contact like an electric charge and which brings death and ruin to anyone who is not protected by a similar charge. Any immediate or indirect contact with this dangerous sacred entity is therefore avoided; and, if it cannot be avoided, some ceremonial is devised to avert the dreaded consequences. The Nubas of East Africa, for instance, 'believe that they would die if they

---

[1] Further examples of these practices will be found in Frazer (1911b, 165–90) in the section upon 'Manslayers tabooed'.

entered the house of their priestly king; however they can evade
the penalty of their intrusion by baring the left shoulder and
getting the king to lay his hand on it.' [Loc. cit.] Here we are
met by the remarkable fact that contact with the king is a rem-
edy and protection against the dangers provoked by contact
with the king. No doubt, however, there is a contrast to be
drawn between the remedial power of a touch made deliberately by the king and the danger which arises if he is touched—
a contrast between a passive and an active relation to the king.

For examples of the healing power of the royal touch there is
no need to resort to savages. The kings of England, in times that
are not yet remote, enjoyed the power of curing scrofula, which
was known accordingly as 'the King's Evil'. Queen Elizabeth
exercised this royal prerogative no less than her successors.
Charles I is said to have cured a hundred patients at a stroke in
1633. But it was after the Restoration of the monarchy under
his dissolute son, Charles II, that the royal cures of scrofula
reached their climax. In the course of his reign he is reputed to
have touched close upon a hundred thousand persons. The
crowd of those in search of cure used to be so great that on one
occasion six or seven of those who came to be healed were
trampled to death. The sceptical William of Orange, who became King of England after the dismissal of the Stuarts, refused
to lend himself to these magical practices. On the only occasion
on which he was persuaded into laying his hands on a patient,
he said to him: 'God give you better health and more sense.'
(Frazer, 1911*a*, **1**, 368–70.)

The stories which follow are evidence of the fearful effects of
active contact made, even unintentionally, with a king or anything belonging to him. 'It once happened that a New Zealand
chief of high rank and great sanctity had left the remains of his
dinner by the wayside. A slave, a stout, hungry fellow, coming
up after the chief had gone, saw the unfinished dinner, and ate
it up without asking questions. Hardly had he finished when he
was informed by a horror-stricken spectator that the food of
which he had eaten was the chief's.' He was a strong, courage-
ous man, but 'no sooner did he hear the fatal news than he was
seized with the most extraordinary convulsions and cramp in
the stomach, which never ceased till he died, about sundown

Taboo and Emotional Ambivalence

the same day'.[1] 'A Maori woman having eaten of some fruit, and being afterwards told that the fruit had been taken from a tabooed place, exclaimed that the spirit of the chief, whose sanctity had been thus profaned, would kill her. This was in the afternoon, and next day by twelve o'clock she was dead.'[2] 'A Maori chief's tinder-box was once the means of killing several persons; for, having been lost by him, and found by some men who used it to light their pipes, they died of fright on learning to whom it had belonged.'[3]

It is not to be wondered at that a need was felt for isolating such dangerous persons as chiefs and priests from the rest of the community—to build a barrier round them which would make them inaccessible. It may begin to dawn on us that this barrier, originally erected for the observance of taboo, exists to this day in the form of court ceremonial.

But perhaps the major part of this taboo upon rulers is not derived from the need for protection *against* them. The second reason for the special treatment of privileged persons—the need to provide protection *for* them against the threat of danger—has had an obvious part in creating taboos and so of giving rise to court etiquette.

The need to protect the king from every possible form of danger follows from his immense importance to his subjects, whether for weal or woe. It is his person which, strictly speaking, regulates the whole course of existence. 'The people have to thank him for the rain and sunshine which foster the fruits of the earth, for the wind which brings ships to their coasts, and even for the solid ground beneath their feet.' (Frazer, 1911*b*, 7.)

These rulers among savage peoples possess a degree of power and a capacity to confer benefits which are an attribute only of gods, and with which at later stages of civilization only the most servile of courtiers would pretend to credit them.

It must strike us as self-contradictory that persons of such unlimited power should need to be protected so carefully from the threat of danger; but that is not the only contradiction shown in

[1] Frazer (1911*b*, 134–5), quoting a Pakeha Maori (1884 [96 f.]).
[2] Frazer (loc. cit.), quoting Brown (1845 [76]).
[3] Frazer (loc. cit.) [quoting Taylor (1870, 164)].

the treatment of royal personages among savage peoples. For these peoples also think it necessary to keep a watch on their king to see that he makes a proper use of his powers; they feel by no means convinced of his good intentions or conscientiousness. Thus an element of distrust may be traced among the reasons for the taboo observances that surround the king. 'The idea', writes Frazer (1911*b*, 7 f.), 'that early kingdoms are despotisms in which the people exist only for the sovereign, is wholly inapplicable to the monarchies we are considering. On the contrary, the sovereign in them exists only for his subjects; his life is only valuable so long as he discharges the duties of his position by ordering the course of nature for his people's benefit. So soon as he fails to do so, the care, the devotion, the religious homage which they had hitherto lavished on him cease and are changed into hatred and contempt; he is dismissed ignominiously, and may be thankful if he escapes with his life. Worshipped as a god one day, he is killed as a criminal the next. But in this changed behaviour of the people there is nothing capricious or inconstant. On the contrary, their conduct is entirely of a piece. If their king is their god, he is or should be also their preserver; and if he will not preserve them, he must make room for another who will. So long, however, as he answers their expectations, there is no limit to the care which they take of him, and which they compel him to take of himself. A king of this sort lives hedged in by a ceremonious etiquette, a network of prohibitions and observances, of which the intention is not to contribute to his dignity, much less to his comfort, but to restrain him from conduct which, by disturbing the harmony of nature, might involve himself, his people, and the universe in one common catastrophe. Far from adding to his comfort, these observances, by trammelling his every act, annihilate his freedom and often render the very life, which it is their object to preserve, a burden and sorrow to him.'

One of the most glaring instances of a sacred ruler being fettered and paralysed in this way by taboo ceremonials is to be found in the mode of life of the Mikado of Japan in earlier centuries. An account written more than two hundred years ago reports that the Mikado 'thinks it would be very prejudicial to his dignity and holiness to touch the ground with his feet; for

44

this reason, when he intends to go anywhere, he must be carried thither on men's shoulders. Much less will they suffer that he should expose his sacred person to the open air, and the sun is not thought worthy to shine on his head. There is such a holiness ascribed to all parts of his body that he dares to cut off neither his hair, nor his beard, nor his nails. However, lest he should grow too dirty, they may clean him in the night when he is asleep; because, they say, that which is taken from his body at that time hath been stolen from him and that such a theft doth not prejudice his holiness or dignity. In ancient times he was obliged to sit on the throne for some hours every morning, with the imperial crown on his head, but to sit altogether like a statue, without stirring either hands or feet, head or eyes, nor indeed any part of his body, because, by this means, it was thought that he could preserve peace and tranquillity in his empire; for if, unfortunately, he turned himself on one side or the other, or if he looked a good while towards any part of his dominions, it was apprehended that war, famine, fire, or some other great misfortune was near at hand to desolate the country.'[1]

Some of the taboos laid upon barbarian kings remind one vividly of the restrictions imposed upon murderers. Thus in West Africa, 'at Shark Point near Cape Padron, in Lower Guinea, lives the priestly king Kukulu, alone in a wood. He may not touch a woman nor leave his house; indeed he may not even quit his chair, in which he is obliged to sleep sitting, for if he lay down no wind would arise and navigation would be stopped. He regulates storms, and in general maintains a wholesome and equable state of the atmosphere.' The same writer says of Loango (in the same part of the world) that the more powerful a king is, the more taboos he is bound to observe.[2] The heir to the throne is also subject to them from infancy; their number increases as he advances in life, till at the moment that he ascends the throne he is positively suffocated by them.

Our space will not allow nor does our interest require us to enter further into a description of the taboos associated with the dignity of kings and priests. I will only add that the principal

[1] Kaempfer (1727 [1, 150]), quoted by Frazer (1911*b*, 3 f.).
[2] Frazer (1911*b*, 5 and 8), quoting Bastian (1874-5 [1, 287 and 355]).

45

part is played in them by restrictions upon freedom of movement and upon diet. Two examples of taboo ceremonials occurring in civilized communities of a far higher level of culture will serve to show, however, what a conservative effect upon ancient usages is exercised by contact with these privileged personages.

The Flamen Dialis, the high priest of Jupiter in ancient Rome, was obliged to observe an extraordinary number of taboos. He 'might not ride or even touch a horse, nor see an army under arms, nor wear a ring which was not broken, nor have a knot on any part of his garments; . . . he might not touch wheaten flour or leavened bread; he might not touch or even name a goat, a dog, raw meat, beans, and ivy; . . . his hair could be cut only by a free man and with a bronze knife, and his hair and nails when cut had to be buried under a lucky tree; . . . he might not touch a dead body; . . . he might not be uncovered in the open air', and so on. 'His wife, the Flaminica, had to observe nearly the same rules, and others of her own besides. She might not ascend more than three steps of the kind of staircase called Greek; at a certain festival she might not comb her hair; the leather of her shoes might not be made from a beast that had died a natural death, but only from one that had been slain or sacrificed; if she heard thunder she was tabooed till she had offered an expiatory sacrifice.' (Frazer, 1911*b*, 13 f.)

The ancient kings of Ireland were subject to a number of exceedingly strange restrictions. If these were obeyed, every kind of blessing would descend upon the country, but if they were violated, disasters of every kind would visit it. A complete list of these taboos is contained in the *Book of Rights*, the two oldest manuscript copies of which date from 1390 and 1418. The prohibitions are of the most detailed character, and refer to specific actions at specific places at specific times: the king, for instance, may not stay in a certain town on a particular day of the week; he may not cross a certain river at a particular hour of the day; he may not encamp for nine days on a certain plain, and so on. (Frazer, 1911*b*, 11 f.)

Among many savage peoples the severity of these taboo restrictions upon priestly kings has led to consequences which have been important historically and are of particular interest from our point of view. The dignity of their position ceased to be an enviable thing, and those who were offered it often took every possible means of escaping it. Thus in Cambodia, where there are kingships of Fire and Water, it is often necessary to force successors into accepting these distinctions. On Niuē or Savage Island, a coral island in the South Pacific, the monarchy actually came to an end because no one could be induced to take over the responsible and dangerous office. 'In some parts of West Africa, when the king dies, a family council is secretly held to determine his successor. He on whom the choice falls is suddenly seized, bound, and thrown into the fetish-house, where he is kept in durance till he consents to accept the crown. Sometimes the heir finds means of evading the honour which it is thought to thrust upon him; a ferocious chief has been known to go about constantly armed, resolute to resist by force any attempt to set him on the throne.'[1] Among the natives of Sierra Leone the objection to accepting the honour of kingship became so great that most tribes were obliged to choose foreigners as their kings.

Frazer (1911*b*, 17–25) attributes to these circumstances the fact that in the course of history there eventually came about a division of the original priestly kingship into a spiritual and a temporal power. Weighed down by the burden of their sacred office, kings became unable to exert their dominance in real affairs and these were left in the hands of inferior but practical persons, who were ready to renounce the honours of kingship. These, then, became the temporal rulers, while spiritual supremacy, deprived of any practical significance, was left to the former taboo kings. It is familiar knowledge how far this hypothesis finds confirmation in the history of old Japan.

If we take a general survey of the relations of primitive men to their rulers, we are left with an expectation that we shall have no great difficulty in advancing from a description of them to a psycho-analytic understanding of them. Those relations are of a complex kind and not free from contradictions. Rulers are allowed great privileges, which coincide exactly with the taboo prohibitions imposed on other people. They are privileged persons: they may do or enjoy precisely what other people are for-

[1] Frazer (1911*b*, 17 f.), quoting Bastian (1874–5 [**1**, 354 and **2**, 9]).

bidden by taboo. As against this freedom, however, we find that they are restricted by other taboos from which common people are exempt. Here we have a first contrast—a contradiction, almost—the fact, that is, of the same individual being both more free and more restricted. Again, they are regarded as possessing extraordinary powers of magic, so that people are afraid of coming into contact with their persons or their property, while on the other hand the most beneficial consequences are expected from that same contact. Here there seems to be another, particularly glaring, contradiction; but, as we have already seen, it is only an apparent one. Contacts originating from the king himself are healing and protective; the dangerous contacts are those effected by common men upon the king or his belongings —probably because they may hint at aggressive impulses. Yet another contradiction, and one not so easily resolved, is to be found in the fact that the ruler is believed to exercise great authority over the forces of Nature, but that he has to be most carefully protected against the threat of danger—as though his own power, which can do so much, cannot do this. The situation is made still more difficult by the fact that the ruler cannot be trusted to make use of his immense powers in the right way, that is, for the benefit of his subjects and for his own protection. Thus people distrust him and feel justified in keeping a watch on him. The etiquette of taboos to which the king's whole life is subjected serves all these protective purposes at once: his own protection from dangers and the protection of his subjects from the dangers with which he threatens them.

It seems plausible to explain the complicated and contradictory attitude of primitive peoples to their rulers in some such way as the following. For superstitious and other reasons, a variety of different impulses find expression in relation to kings; and each of these impulses is developed to an extreme point without regard to the others. This gives rise to contradictions—by which, incidentally, a savage intellect is as little disturbed as is a highly civilized one when it comes to such matters as religion or 'loyalty'.

So far so good; but the technique of psycho-analysis allows us to go into the question further and to enter more into the details of these various impulses. If we submit the recorded facts to analysis, as though they formed part of the symptoms presented by a neurosis, our starting-point must be the excessive apprehensiveness and solicitude which is put forward as the reason for the taboo ceremonials. The occurrence of excessive solicitude of this kind is very common in neuroses, and especially in obsessional neuroses, with which our comparison is chiefly drawn. We have come to understand its origin quite clearly. It appears wherever, in addition to a predominant feeling of affection, there is also a contrary, but unconscious, current of hostility—a state of affairs which represents a typical instance of an ambivalent emotional attitude. The hostility is then shouted down, as it were, by an excessive intensification of the affection, which is expressed as solicitude and becomes compulsive, because it might otherwise be inadequate to perform its task of keeping the unconscious contrary current of feeling under repression. Every psychoanalyst knows from experience with what certainty this explanation of solicitous over-affection is found to apply even in the most unlikely circumstances—in cases, for instance, of attachments between a mother and child or between a devoted married couple. If we now apply this to the case of privileged persons, we shall realize that alongside of the veneration, and indeed idolization, felt towards them, there is in the unconscious an opposing current of intense hostility; that, in fact, as we expected, we are faced by a situation of emotional ambivalence. The distrust which provides one of the unmistakable elements in kingly taboos would thus be another, more direct, expression of the same unconscious hostility. Indeed, owing to the variety of outcomes of a conflict of this kind which are reached among different peoples, we are not at a loss for examples in which the existence of this hostility is still more obviously shown. 'The savage Timmes of Sierra Leone', we learn from Frazer,[1] 'who elect their king, reserve to themselves the right of beating him on the eve of his coronation; and they avail themselves of this constitutional privilege with such hearty goodwill that sometimes the unhappy monarch does not long survive his elevation to the throne. Hence when the leading chiefs have a spite at a man and wish to rid themselves of him, they elect him king.' Even in glaring instances like this, however, the hostility is not admitted as such, but masquerades as a ceremonial.

[1] Frazer (1911*b*, 18), quoting Zweifel and Moustier (1880 [28]).

Totem and Taboo

Another side of the attitude of primitive peoples towards their rulers recalls a procedure which is common in neuroses generally but comes into the open in what are known as delusions of persecution. The importance of one particular person is immensely exaggerated and his absolute power is magnified to the most improbable degree, in order that it may be easier to make him responsible for everything disagreeable that the patient may experience. Savages are really behaving in just the same way with their kings when they ascribe to them power over rain and sunshine, wind and weather, and then depose them or kill them because Nature disappoints their hopes of a successful hunt or a rich harvest. The model upon which paranoiacs base their delusions of persecution is the relation of a child to his father. A son's picture of his father is habitually clothed with excessive powers of this kind, and it is found that distrust of the father is intimately linked with admiration for him. When a paranoiac turns the figure of one of his associates into a 'persecutor', he is raising him to the rank of a father: he is putting him into a position in which he can blame him for all his misfortunes. Thus this second analogy between savages and neurotics gives us a glimpse of the truth that much of a savage's attitude to his ruler is derived from a child's infantile attitude to his father.

But the strongest support for our effort to equate taboo prohibitions with neurotic symptoms is to be found in the taboo ceremonials themselves, the effect of which upon the position of royalty has already been discussed. These ceremonials unmistakably reveal their double meaning and their derivation from ambivalent impulses, as soon as we are ready to allow that the results which they bring about were intended from the first. The taboo does not only pick out the king and exalt him above all common mortals, it also makes his existence a torment and an intolerable burden and reduces him to a bondage far worse than that of his subjects. Here, then, we have an exact counterpart of the obsessional act in the neurosis, in which the suppressed impulse and the impulse that suppresses it find simultaneous and common satisfaction. The obsessional act is *ostensibly* a protection against the prohibited act; but *actually*, in our view, it is a repetition of it. The 'ostensibly' applies to the *conscious* part of the mind, and the 'actually' to the *unconscious* part. In exactly the same way, the ceremonial taboo of kings is *ostensibly* the highest honour and protection for them, while *actually* it is a punishment for their exaltation, a revenge taken on them by their subjects. The experiences of Sancho Panza (as described by Cervantes) when he was Governor of his island convinced him that this view of court ceremonial was the only one that met the case. If we could hear the views of modern kings and rulers on the subject, we might find that there were many others who agreed with him.

The question of why the emotional attitude towards rulers includes such a powerful unconscious element of hostility raises a very interesting problem, but one that lies outside the limits of the present study. I have already hinted at the fact that the child's complex of emotions towards his father—the father-complex—has a bearing on the subject, and I may add that more information on the early history of the kingship would throw a decisive light on it. Frazer (1911a) has put forward impressive reasons, though, as he himself admits, not wholly conclusive ones, for supposing that the earliest kings were foreigners who, after a brief reign, were sacrificed with solemn festivities as representatives of the deity. It is possible that the course taken by the evolution of kings may also have had an influence upon the myths of Christendom.

(c) The Taboo upon the Dead

We know that the dead are powerful rulers; but we may perhaps be surprised when we learn that they are treated as enemies.

The taboo upon the dead is—if I may revert to the simile of infection—especially virulent among most primitive peoples. It is manifested, in the first instance, in the consequences that follow contact with the dead and in the treatment of mourners.

Among the Maoris anyone who had handled a corpse or taken any part in its burial was in the highest degree unclean and was almost cut off from intercourse with his fellow-men, or, as we might put it, was boycotted. He could not enter any house, or come into contact with any person or thing without infecting them. He might not even touch food with his hands, which, owing to their uncleanness, had become quite useless. 'Food would be set for him on the ground, and he would then sit or kneel down, and, with his hands carefully held behind his back, would gnaw at it as best he could. In some cases he would be fed by another person, who with outstretched arm contrived to do it without touching the tabooed man; but the feeder was himself subjected to many severe restrictions, little less onerous than those which were imposed upon the other. In almost every populous village there lived a degraded wretch, the lowest of the low, who earned a sorry pittance by thus waiting upon the defiled.' He alone was allowed 'to associate at arm's length with one who had paid the last offices . . . to the dead. And when, the dismal term of his seclusion being over, the mourner was about to mix with his fellows once more, all the dishes he had used in his seclusion were diligently smashed, and all the garments he had worn were carefully thrown away.' [Frazer, 1911*b*, 138 f.]

The taboo observances after bodily contact with the dead are the same over the whole of Polynesia, Melanesia and a part of Africa. Their most regular feature is the prohibition against those who have had such contact touching food themselves, and the consequent necessity for their being fed by other people. It is a remarkable fact that in Polynesia (though the report may perhaps refer only to Hawaii) priestly kings were subject to the same restriction while performing their sacred functions.[1] The case of the taboo upon the dead in Tonga offers a specially clear instance of the way in which the degree of prohibition varies according to the taboo power of the person upon whom the taboo is imposed. Thus anyone who touches a dead chief is unclean for ten months; but if he himself is a chief he is only tabooed for three, four, or five months according to the rank of the dead man; but if the dead man were the 'great divine chief', even the greatest chief would be tabooed for ten months. These savages believe firmly that anyone who violates the taboo ordinances is bound to fall ill and die; indeed they believe it so firmly that, in the opinion of an observer, 'no native ever made an experiment to prove the contrary'.[2]

[1] Frazer (loc. cit.) [quoting Ellis (1832–6, 4, 388)].
[2] Frazer (1911*b*, 140), quoting Mariner (1818 [1, 141]).

Taboo and Emotional Ambivalence

Essentially the same prohibitions (though from our point of view they are more interesting) apply to those who have been in contact with the dead only in a metaphorical sense: the dead person's mourning relations, widowers and widows. The observances that we have so far mentioned may seem merely to give characteristic expression to the virulence of the taboo and its contagious power. But those which now follow give us a hint at the *reasons* for the taboo—both the ostensible ones and what we must regard as the deep-lying real ones.

'Among the Shuswap of British Columbia widows and widowers in mourning are secluded and forbidden to touch their own head or body; the cups and cooking vessels which they use may be used by no one else. . . . No hunter would come near such mourners, for their presence is unlucky. If their shadow were to fall on anyone, he would be taken ill at once. They employ thorn-bushes for bed and pillow . . . and thorn-bushes are also laid all around their beds.'[1] This last measure is designed to keep the dead person's ghost at a distance. The same purpose is shown still more clearly in the usage reported from another North American tribe which provides that, after her husband's death, 'a widow would wear a breech-cloth made of dry bunch-grass for several days to prevent her husband's ghost having intercourse with her.'[2] This suggests that contact 'in a metaphorical sense' is after all understood as being bodily contact, for the dead man's ghost does not leave his relations and does not cease to 'hover' round them during the time of mourning.

'Among the Agutainos, who inhabit Palawan, one of the Philippine Islands, a widow may not leave her hut for seven or eight days after the death; and even then she may only go out at an hour when she is not likely to meet anybody, for whoever looks upon her dies a sudden death. To prevent this fatal catastrophe, the widow knocks with a wooden peg on the trees as she goes along, thus warning people of her dangerous proximity; and the very trees on which she knocks soon die.'[3] The nature of the danger feared from a widow such as this is made plain by another example. 'In the Mekeo district of British New Guinea

[1] [Frazer (1911*b*, 142), quoting Boas (1890, 643 f.).]
[2] [Frazer (1911*b*, 143), quoting Teit (1900, 332 f.).]
[3] [Frazer (1911*b*, 144), quoting Blumentritt (1891, 182).]

a widower loses all his civil rights and becomes a social outcast, an object of fear and horror, shunned by all. He may not cultivate a garden, nor show himself in public, nor walk on the roads and paths. Like a wild beast he must skulk in the long grass and the bushes; and if he sees or hears anyone coming, especially a woman, he must hide behind a tree or a thicket.'[1] This last hint makes it easy to trace the origin of the dangerous character of widowers or widows to the danger of *temptation*. A man who has lost his wife must resist a desire to find a substitute for her; a widow must fight against the same wish and is moreover liable, being without a lord and master, to arouse the desires of other men. Substitutive satisfactions of such a kind run counter to the sense of mourning and they would inevitably kindle the ghost's wrath.[2]

One of the most puzzling, but at the same time instructive, usages in connection with mourning is the prohibition against uttering the name of the dead person. This custom is extremely widespread, it is expressed in a variety of ways and has had important consequences. It is found not only among the Australians and Polynesians (who usually show us taboo observances in the best state of preservation), but also among 'peoples so widely separated from each other as the Samoyeds of Siberia and the Todas of southern India; the Mongols of Tartary and the Tuaregs of the Sahara; the Ainos of Japan and the Akamba and Nandi of central Africa; the Tinguianes of the Philippines and the inhabitants of the Nicobar Islands, of Borneo, of Madagascar, and of Tasmania.' (Frazer, 1911*b*, 353.) In some of these cases the prohibition and its consequences last only during the period of mourning, in others they are permanent; but it seems invariably to diminish in strictness with the passage of time.

The avoidance of the name of a dead person is as a rule enforced with extreme severity. Thus in some South American tribes it is regarded as a deadly insult to the survivors to mention

---

[1] [Frazer (1911*b*, 144), quoting Guis (1902, 208 f.).]

[2] The patient whose 'impossibilities' I compared with taboos earlier in this paper (see page 28) told me that whenever she met anyone dressed in mourning in the street she was filled with indignation: such people, she thought, should be forbidden to go out.

the name of a dead relative in their presence, and the punishment for it is not less than that laid down for murder. (Ibid., 352.) It is not easy at first to see why the mention of the name should be regarded with such horror; but the dangers involved have given rise to a whole number of methods of evasion which are interesting and important in various ways. Thus the Masai in East Africa resort to the device of changing the dead man's name immediately after his death; he may then be mentioned freely under his new name while all the restrictions remain attached to the old one. This seems to presuppose that the dead man's ghost does not know and will not get to know his new name. [Ibid., 354.] The Adelaide and Encounter Bay tribes of South Australia are so consistently careful that after a death everyone bearing the same name as the dead man's, or a very similar one, changes it for another. [Ibid., 355.] In some instances, as for instance among certain tribes in Victoria and in North-West America, this is carried a step further, and after a death all the dead person's relations change their names, irrespective of any similarity in their sound. [Ibid., 357.] Indeed, among the Guaycurus in Paraguay, when a death had taken place, the chief used to change the name of every member of the tribe; and 'from that moment everybody remembered his new name just as if he had borne it all his life'.[1]

Moreover, if the name of the dead man happens to be the same as that of an animal or common object, some tribes think it necessary to give these animals or objects new names, so that the use of the former names shall not recall the dead man to memory. This usage leads to a perpetual change of vocabulary, which causes much difficulty to the missionaries, especially when such changes are permanent. In the seven years which the missionary Dobrizhoffer spent among the Abipones of Paraguay, 'the native word for jaguar was changed thrice, and the words for crocodile, thorn, and the slaughter of cattle underwent similar though less varied vicissitudes'.[2] The dread of uttering a dead person's name extends, indeed, to an avoidance of the mention of anything in which the dead man played a

[1] Frazer (1911*b*, 357), quoting an old Spanish observer [Lozano (1733, 70)].
[2] Frazer (1911*b*, 360), quoting Dobrizhoffer [1784, 2, 301].

part; and an important consequence of this process of suppression is that these peoples possess no tradition and no historical memory, so that any research into their early history is faced by the greatest difficulties. [Ibid., 362 f.] A number of these primitive races have, however, adopted compensatory usages which revive the names of dead persons after a long period of mourning by giving them to children, who are thus regarded as reincarnations of the dead. [Ibid., 364 f.]

This taboo upon names will seem less puzzling if we bear in mind the fact that savages regard a name as an essential part of a man's personality and as an important possession: they treat words in every sense as things. As I have pointed out elsewhere [Freud, 1905b, Chap. IV], our own children do the same. They are never ready to accept a similarity between two words as having no meaning; they consistently assume that if two things are called by similar-sounding names this must imply the existence of some deep-lying point of agreement between them. Even a civilized adult may be able to infer from certain peculiarities in his own behaviour that he is not so far removed as he may have thought from attributing importance to proper names, and that his own name has become to a very remarkable extent bound up with his personality. So, too, psycho-analytic practice comes upon frequent confirmations of this in the evidence it finds of the importance of names in unconscious mental activities.[1]

As was only to be expected, obsessional neurotics behave exactly like savages in relation to names. Like other neurotics, they show a high degree of 'complexive sensitiveness'[2] in regard to uttering or hearing particular words and names; and their attitude towards their own names imposes numerous, and often serious, inhibitions upon them. One of these taboo patients of my acquaintance had adopted a rule against writing her own name, for fear that it might fall into the hands of someone who would then be in possession of a portion of her personality. She was obliged to fight with convulsive loyalty against the temptations to which her imagination subjected her, and so forbade

[1] Cf. Stekel [1911] and Abraham [1912].
[2] [*Komplexempfindlichkeit*—a term used by Jung in connection with his word association experiments.]

herself 'to surrender any part of her person'. This included in the first place her name, and later extended to her handwriting, till finally she gave up writing altogether.

We shall no longer feel surprised, therefore, at savages regarding the name of a dead person as a portion of his personality and making it subject to the relevant taboo. So, too, uttering the name of a dead person is clearly a derivative of having contact with him. We may therefore turn to the wider problem of why such contact is submitted to so strict a taboo.

The most obvious explanation would point to horror roused by dead bodies and by the changes which quickly become visible in them. Some part must also be played in the matter by mourning for the dead person, since it must be a motive force in everything relating to him. But horror at the corpse clearly does not account for all the details of the taboo observances, and mourning cannot explain why the uttering of the dead man's name is an insult to his survivors. Mourning, on the contrary, tends to be preoccupied with the dead man, to dwell upon his memory and to preserve it as long as possible. Something other than mourning must be held responsible for the peculiarities of the taboo usages, something which has very different purposes in view. It is precisely the taboo upon names that gives us the clue to this unknown motive; and if the usages alone did not tell us, we should learn it from what the mourning savages say to us themselves.

For they make no disguise of the fact that they are *afraid* of the presence or of the return of the dead person's ghost; and they perform a great number of ceremonies to keep him at a distance or drive him off.[1] They feel that to utter his name is equivalent to invoking him and will quickly be followed by his presence.[2] And accordingly they do everything they can to avoid any such evocation. They disguise themselves so that the ghost shall not recognize them,[3] or they change his name or

---

[1] Frazer (1911*b* 353) mentions the Tuaregs of the Sahara as an example of this explanation being given by the savages themselves.

[2] Subject, perhaps, to the condition that some of his bodily remains are still in existence. (Ibid., 372.)

[3] In the Nicobar Islands. (Ibid., 358.)

their own; they are furious with reckless strangers who by uttering the ghost's name incite him against the survivors. It is impossible to escape the conclusion that, in the words of Wundt
(1906, 49), they are victims to a fear of 'the dead man's soul
which has become a demon'. Here, then, we seem to have
found a confirmation of Wundt's view, which, as we have already seen (p. 24), considers that the essence of taboo is a fear of
demons.

This theory is based on a supposition so extraordinary that it
seems at first sight incredible: the supposition, namely, that a
dearly loved relative at the moment of his death changes into a
demon, from whom his survivors can expect nothing but hostility and against whose evil desires they must protect themselves by every possible means. Nevertheless, almost all the
authorities are at one in attributing these views to primitive
peoples. Westermarck, who, in my opinion, takes far too little
notice of taboo in his book on *The Origin and Development of the
Moral Ideas*, actually writes in his chapter on 'Regard for the
Dead': 'Generally speaking, my collection of facts has led me to
the conclusion that the dead are more commonly regarded as
enemies than friends, and that Professor Jevons and Mr. Grant
Allen are mistaken in their assertion that, according to early
beliefs, the malevolence of the dead is for the most part directed
against strangers only, whereas they exercise a fatherly care
over the lives and fortunes of their descendants and fellow
clansmen.'[1]

In an interesting volume, Rudolf Kleinpaul (1898) has used
the remnants among civilized races of the ancient belief in

[1] Westermarck (1906–8, **2**, 532 ff.). In his footnotes and in the section
of the text which follows, the author gives copious confirmatory evidence,
often of a highly characteristic sort. For instance: 'Among the Maoris
the nearest and most beloved relatives were supposed to have their
natures changed by death, and to become malignant, even towards those
they formerly loved. [Quoting Taylor (1870, 18).] . . . Australian
natives believed that a deceased person is malevolent for a long time
after death, and the more nearly related the more he is feared. [Quoting
Fraser (1892, 80).] . . . According to ideas prevalent among the Central
Eskimo, the dead are at first malevolent spirits who frequently roam
around the villages, causing sickness and mischief and killing men by
their touch; but subsequently they are supposed to attain rest and are
no longer feared. [Quoting Boas (1888, 591).]'

spirits to throw light on the relation between the living and the dead. He, too, reaches the final conclusion that the dead, filled with a lust for murder, sought to drag the living in their train. The dead slew; and the skeleton which we use to-day to picture the dead stands for the fact that they themselves were slayers. The living did not feel safe from the attacks of the dead till there was a sheet of water between them. That is why men liked to bury the dead on islands or on the farther side of rivers; and that, in turn, is the origin of such phrases as 'Here and in the Beyond'. Later, the malignity of the dead diminished and was restricted to special categories which had a particular right to feel resentment—such as murdered men, for instance, who in the form of evil spirits went in pursuit of their murderers, or brides, who had died with their desires unsatisfied. But originally, says Kleinpaul, *all* of the dead were vampires, all of them had a grudge against the living and sought to injure them and rob them of their lives. It was from corpses that the concept of evil spirits first arose.

The hypothesis that after their death those most beloved were transformed into demons clearly raises further questions. What was it that induced primitive men to attribute such a change of feeling to those who had been dear to them? Why did they make them into demons? Westermarck (1906–8, **2**, 534 f.) is of the opinion that these questions can be answered easily. 'Death is commonly regarded as the gravest of all misfortunes; hence the dead are believed to be exceedingly dissatisfied with their fate. According to primitive ideas a person only dies if he is killed— by magic if not by force—and such a death naturally tends to make the soul revengeful and ill-tempered. It is envious of the living and is longing for the company of its old friends; no wonder, then, that it sends them diseases to cause their death. . . . But the notion that the disembodied soul is on the whole a malicious being . . . is also, no doubt, intimately connected with the instinctive fear of the dead, which is in its turn the outcome of the fear of death.'

The study of psycho-neurotic disorders suggests a more comprehensive explanation, which at the same time covers that put forward by Westermarck.

Totem and Taboo

When a wife has lost her husband or a daughter her mother, it not infrequently happens that the survivor is overwhelmed by tormenting doubts (to which we give the name of 'obsessive self-reproaches') as to whether she may not herself have been responsible for the death of this cherished being through some act of carelessness or neglect. No amount of recollection of the care she lavished on the sufferer, no amount of objective disproof of the accusation, serves to bring the torment to an end. It may be regarded as a pathological form of mourning, and with the passage of time it gradually dies away. The psychoanalytic investigation of such cases has revealed the secret motives of the disorder. We find that in a certain sense these obsessive self-reproaches are justified, and that this is why they are proof against contradictions and protests. It is not that the mourner was really responsible for the death or was really guilty of neglect, as the self-reproaches declare to be the case. None the less there was something in her—a wish that was unconscious to herself—which would not have been dissatisfied by the occurrence of death and which might actually have brought it about if it had had the power. And after death *has* occurred, it is against this unconscious wish that the reproaches are a reaction. In almost every case where there is an intense emotional attachment to a particular person we find that behind the tender love there is a concealed hostility in the unconscious. This is the classical example, the prototype, of the ambivalence of human emotions. This ambivalence is present to a greater or less amount in the innate disposition of everyone; normally, there is not so much of it as to produce the obsessive self-reproaches we are considering. Where, however, it is copiously present in the disposition, it will manifest itself precisely in the subject's relation to those of whom he is most fond, in the place, in fact, where one would least expect to find it. It must be supposed that the presence of a particularly large amount of this original emotional ambivalence is characteristic of the disposition of obsessional neurotics—whom I have so often brought up for comparison in this discussion upon taboo.

We have now discovered a motive which can explain the idea that the souls of those who have just died are transformed into demons and the necessity felt by survivors to protect themselves by taboos against their hostility. Let us suppose that the emotional life of primitive peoples is characterized by an amount of ambivalence as great as that which we are led by the findings of psycho-analysis to attribute to obsessional patients. It then becomes easy to understand how after a painful bereavement savages should be obliged to produce a reaction against the hostility latent in their unconscious similar to that expressed as obsessive self-reproach in the case of neurotics. But this hostility, distressingly felt in the unconscious as satisfaction over the death, is differently dealt with among primitive peoples. The defence against it takes the form of displacing it on to the object of the hostility, on to the dead themselves. This defensive procedure, which is a common one both in normal and in pathological mental life, is known as a *'projection'*. The survivor thus denies that he has ever harboured any hostile feelings against the dead loved one; the soul of the dead harbours them instead and seeks to put them into action during the whole period of mourning. In spite of the successful defence which the survivor achieves by means of projection, his emotional reaction shows the characteristics of punishment and remorse, for he is the subject of fears and submits to renunciations and restrictions, though these are in part disguised as measures of protection against the hostile demon. Once again, therefore, we find that the taboo has grown up on the basis of an ambivalent emotional attitude. The taboo upon the dead arises, like the others, from the contrast between conscious pain and unconscious satisfaction over the death that has occurred. Since such is the origin of the ghost's resentment, it follows naturally that the survivors who have the most to fear will be those who were formerly its nearest and dearest.

In this respect taboo observances, like neurotic symptoms, have a double sense. On the one hand, in their restrictive character, they are expressions of mourning; but on the other hand they clearly betray—what they seek to conceal—hostility against the dead disguised as self-defence. We have already learned that certain taboos arise out of fear of temptation. The fact that a dead man is helpless is bound to act as an encouragement to the survivor to give free rein to his hostile passions, and that temptation must be countered by a prohibition.

Totem and Taboo

Westermarck is right in insisting that savages draw no distinction between violent and natural death. In the view of unconscious thinking, a man who has died a natural death is a murdered man: evil wishes have killed him.[1] Anyone who investigates the origin and significance of dreams of the death of loved relatives (of parents or brothers or sisters) will be able to convince himself that dreamers, children and savages are at one in their attitude towards the dead—an attitude based upon emotional ambivalence.[2]

At the beginning of this essay [p. 24] disagreement was expressed with Wundt's opinion that the essence of taboo was a fear of demons. Yet we have now assented to an explanation that derives the taboo upon the dead from a fear of the soul of the dead person transformed into a demon. The apparent contradiction can easily be resolved. It is true that we have accepted the presence of demons, but not as something ultimate and psychologically unanalysable. We have succeeded, as it were, in getting behind the demons, for we have explained them as projections of hostile feelings harboured by the survivors against the dead.

Both of the two sets of feelings (the affectionate and the hostile), which, as we have good reason to believe, exist towards the dead person, seek to take effect at the time of the bereavement, as mourning and as satisfaction. There is bound to be a conflict between these two contrary feelings; and, since one of the two, the hostility, is wholly or for the greater part unconscious, the outcome of the conflict cannot be to subtract, as it were, the feeling with the lesser intensity from that with the greater and to establish the remainder in consciousness—as occurs, for instance, when one forgives a slight that one has received from someone of whom one is fond. The process is dealt with instead by the special psychical mechanism known in psycho-analysis, as I have said, by the name of 'projection'. The hostility, of which the survivors know nothing and moreover wish to know nothing, is ejected from internal perception into the external world, and thus detached from them and pushed

[1] Cf. the next essay in this volume.
[2] [Cf. Freud: *The Interpretation of Dreams* (1900), English translation, 1932, 242 ff.]

on to someone else. It is no longer true that they are rejoicing to be rid of the dead man; on the contrary, they are mourning for him; but, strange to say, *he* has turned into a wicked demon ready to gloat over their misfortunes and eager to kill them. It then becomes necessary for them, the survivors, to defend themselves against this evil enemy; they are relieved of pressure from within, but have only exchanged it for oppression from without.

It cannot be disputed that this process of projection, which turns a dead man into a malignant enemy, is able to find support in any real acts of hostility on his part that may be recollected and felt as a grudge against him: his severity, his love of power, his unfairness, or whatever else may form the background of even the tenderest of human relationships. But it cannot be such a simple matter as that. This factor alone cannot explain the creation of demons by projection. The faults of the dead no doubt provide a part of the explanation of the survivors' hostility; but they would not operate in this way unless the survivors had first developed hostility on their own account. The moment of death, moreover, would certainly seem to be a most inappropriate occasion for recalling any justifiable grounds of complaint that might exist. It is impossible to escape the fact that the true determining factor is invariably *unconscious* hostility. A hostile current of feeling such as this against a person's nearest and dearest relatives may remain latent during their lifetime, that is, its existence may not be betrayed to consciousness either directly or through some substitute. But when they die this is no longer possible and the conflict becomes acute. The mourning which derives from an intensification of the affectionate feelings becomes on the one hand more impatient of the latent hostility and, on the other hand, will not allow it to give rise to any sense of satisfaction. Accordingly, there follow the repression of the unconscious hostility by the method of projection and the construction of the ceremonial which gives expression to the fear of being punished by the demons. When in course of time the mourning runs its course, the conflict grows less acute, so that the taboo upon the dead is able to diminish in severity or sink into oblivion.

Totem and Taboo

(4)

Having thus explained the basis of the exceedingly instructive taboo upon the dead, we must not omit to add a few remarks that may help to increase our understanding of taboo in general.

The projection of unconscious hostility on to demons in the case of the taboo upon the dead is only a single instance of a number of processes to which the greatest influence must be attributed in the shaping of the primitive mind. In the case we have been dealing with, projection served the purpose of dealing with an emotional conflict; and it is employed in the same way in a large number of psychical situations that lead to neuroses. But projection was not created for the purpose of defence; it also occurs where there is no conflict. The projection outwards of internal perceptions is a primitive mechanism, to which, for instance, our sense perceptions are subject, and which therefore normally plays a very large part in determining the form taken by our external world. Under conditions whose nature has not yet been sufficiently established, internal perceptions of emotional and intellective processes can be projected outwards in the same way as sense perceptions; they are thus employed for building up the external world, though they should by rights remain part of the *internal* world. This may have some genetic connection with the fact that the function of attention was originally directed not towards the internal world but towards the stimuli that stream in from the external world, and that that function's only information upon endopsychic processes was received from feelings of pleasure and unpleasure. It was not until a language of abstract thought had been developed, that is to say, not until the sensory residues of verbal presentations had been linked to the internal processes, that the latter themselves gradually became capable of being perceived. Before that, owing to the projection outwards of internal perceptions, primitive men arrived at a picture of the external world which we, with our intensified conscious perception, have now to translate back into psychology.

The projection of their own evil impulses into demons is only one portion of a system which constituted the *Weltanschauung* [view of the universe] of primitive peoples, and which we shall come to know as 'animism' in the following essay. There we shall have to investigate that system's psychological characteristics, and we shall do so once again by reference to the similar systems which we find constructed by neurotics. For the moment I will only say that the prototype of all such systems is what we have termed the 'secondary revision' of the content of dreams.[1] And we must not forget that, at and after the stage at which systems are constructed, two sets of reasons can be assigned for every psychical event that is consciously judged—one set belonging to the system and the other set real but unconscious.[2]

Wundt (1906, 129) remarks that 'among the activities attributed by myths all over the world to demons, the harmful predominate, so that in popular belief bad demons are clearly older than good ones'. It is quite possible that the whole concept of demons was derived from the important relation of the living to the dead. The ambivalence inherent in that relation was expressed in the subsequent course of human development by the fact that, from the same root, it gave rise to two completely opposed psychical structures: on the one hand fear of demons and ghosts and on the other hand veneration of ancestors.[3] The fact that demons are always regarded as the spirits of those who have died *recently* shows better than anything the influence of mourning on the origin of the belief in demons. Mourning has a quite specific psychical task to perform: its function is to detach the survivors' memories and hopes from the dead. When this has been achieved, the pain grows less and with it the remorse and self-reproaches and consequently the fear of the demon as

[1] [Cf. Freud: *The Interpretation of Dreams* (1900), English translation, 1932, 451 ff.]

[2] [Further explained below, p. 94f.] The projected creations of primitive men resemble the personifications constructed by creative writers; for the latter externalize in the form of separate individuals the opposing instinctual impulses struggling within them.

[3] In the course of psycho-analyses of neurotics who suffer (or who suffered in their childhood) from fear of ghosts, it is often possible to show without much difficulty that the ghosts are disguises for the patient's parents. Cf. in this connection a paper upon 'Sexual Ghosts' by Haeberlin (1912). Here the person concerned was not the subject's parent (who was dead) but someone else of erotic significance to him.

well. And the same spirits who to begin with were feared as demons may now expect to meet with friendlier treatment, they are revered as ancestors and appeals are made to them for help.

If we follow the changing relations between survivors and the dead through the course of ages, it becomes obvious that there has been an extraordinary diminution in ambivalence. It is now quite easy to keep down the unconscious hostility to the dead (though its existence can still be traced) without any particular expenditure of psychical energy. Where, in earlier times, satisfied hatred and pained affection fought each other, we now find that a kind of scar has been formed in the shape of piety, which declares '*de mortuis nil nisi bonum*'. It is only neurotics whose mourning for the loss of those dear to them is still troubled by obsessive self-reproaches—the secret of which is revealed by psycho-analysis as the old emotional ambivalence. We need not discuss here how this alteration came about or how much share in it is due to a constitutional modification and how much to a real improvement in family relations. But this example suggests the probability that the psychical impulses of primitive peoples were characterized by a higher amount of ambivalence than is to be found in modern civilized man. It is to be supposed that as this ambivalence diminished, taboo (a symptom of the ambivalence and a compromise between the two conflicting impulses) slowly disappeared.[1] Neurotics, who are obliged to reproduce the struggle and the taboo resulting from it, may be said to have inherited an archaic constitution as an atavistic vestige; the need to compensate for this at the behest of civilization is what drives them to their immense expenditure of mental energy.

And here we may recall the obscure and puzzling statement by Wundt on the double meaning of the word taboo: 'sacred' and 'unclean'. (See above [p. 25].) Originally, according to him, the word did not possess these two meanings, but described 'what is demonic', 'what may not be touched', thus stressing an important characteristic common to both the extreme concepts. The persistence, however (he added), of this common charac-

[1] [The last two sentences are in spaced type in the original.]

teristic was evidence that the ground covered by the two—the sacred and the unclean—was originally one and did not become differentiated until later.

Our discussions, on the contrary, lead us to the simple conclusion that the word 'taboo' had a double meaning from the very first and that it was used to designate a particular kind of ambivalence and whatever arose from it. 'Taboo' is itself an ambivalent word; and one feels on looking back that the well-attested meaning of the word should alone have made it possible to infer—what has actually been arrived at as a result of extensive researches—that the prohibitions of taboo are to be understood as consequences of an emotional ambivalence. Study of the earliest languages has taught us that there were once many such words, which expressed contrary ideas and in a sense (though not in quite the same sense as the word 'taboo') were ambivalent.[1] Slight modifications in the pronunciation of the antithetical 'primal word' made it possible subsequently to give separate verbal expression to the two contrary ideas which were originally combined in it.

The word 'taboo' met with a different fate. As the importance of the ambivalence denoted by it diminished, the word itself, or rather the words analogous to it, fell out of use. I hope to be able, in a later connection, to make it probable that a definite historical chain of events is concealed behind the fate of this concept: that the word was at first attached to certain quite specific human relations which were characterized by great emotional ambivalence, and that its use then spread on to other analogous relations.

If I am not mistaken, the explanation of taboo also throws light on the nature and origin of *conscience*. It is possible, without any stretching of the sense of the terms, to speak of a taboo conscience or, after a taboo has been violated, of a taboo sense of guilt. Taboo conscience is probably the earliest form in which the phenomenon of conscience is met with.

For what is 'conscience'? On the evidence of language it is related to that of which one is 'most certainly conscious'. In-

[1] Cf. my review of Abel's 'Antithetical Sense of Primal Words' [Freud, 1910].

67

deed, in some languages the words for 'conscience' and 'conscious' can scarcely be distinguished.[1]

Conscience is the internal perception of the rejection of a particular wish operating within us. The stress, however, is upon the fact that this rejection has no need to appeal to anything else for support, that it is quite 'certain of itself'. This is even clearer in the case of consciousness of guilt—the perception of the internal condemnation of an act by which we have carried out a particular wish. To put forward any reason for this would seem superfluous: anyone who has a conscience must feel within him the justification for the condemnation, must feel the self-reproach for the act that has been carried out. This same characteristic is to be seen in the savage's attitude towards taboo. It is a command issued by conscience; any violation of it produces a fearful sense of guilt which follows as a matter of course and of which the origin is unknown.[2]

Thus it seems probable that conscience too arose, on a basis of emotional ambivalence, from quite specific human relations to which this ambivalence was attached; and that it arose under the conditions which we have shown to apply in the case of taboo and of obsessional neurosis—namely, that one of the opposing feelings involved shall be unconscious and kept under repression by the compulsive domination of the other one. This conclusion is supported by several things we have learnt from the analysis of neuroses.

In the first place, we have found that a feature in the character of obsessional neurotics is a scrupulous conscientiousness which is a symptom reacting against the temptation lurking in their unconscious. If their illness becomes more acute, they develop a sense of guilt of the most intense degree. In fact, one

[1] [E.g. the French *'conscience'*, which has both meanings. The German word for 'conscience' is *'Gewissen'*, which contains the same root as such words as *'wissen'*, 'to know', and *'bewusst'*, 'conscious', as well as the word actually used for comparison in this paragraph and the next, *'gewiss'*, 'certain' or 'known with certainty'.]

[2] The sense of guilt in the case of taboos is not in the least diminished if the violation occurs unwittingly. (Cf. the instances above [p. 42 f.].) An interesting parallel is found in Greek mythology: the guilt of Œdipus was not palliated by the fact that he incurred it without his knowledge and even against his intention.

may venture to say that if we cannot trace the origin of the sense of guilt in obsessional neurotics, there can be no hope of our *ever* tracing it. This task can be directly achieved in the case of individual neurotic patients, and we may rely upon reaching a similar solution by inference in the case of primitive peoples.

In the second place, we cannot help being struck by the fact that a sense of guilt has about it much of the nature of anxiety: we could describe it without any misgivings as 'dread of conscience'. But the anxiety points to unconscious sources. The psychology of the neuroses has taught us that, if wishful impulses are repressed, their libido is transformed into anxiety. And this reminds us that there is something unknown and unconscious in connection with the sense of guilt, namely the reasons for the act of repudiation. The character of anxiety that is inherent in the sense of guilt corresponds to this unknown factor.[1]

Since taboos are mainly expressed in prohibitions, the underlying presence of a *positive* current of desire may occur to us as something quite obvious and calling for no lengthy proofs based on the analogy of the neuroses. For, after all, there is no need to prohibit something that no one desires to do, and a thing that is forbidden with the greatest emphasis must be a thing that is desired. If we were to apply this plausible thesis to our primitive peoples, we should be led to the conclusion that some of their strongest temptations were to kill their kings and priests, to commit incest, to maltreat the dead, and so on—which seems scarcely probable. And we should be met with the most positive contradiction if we were to apply the same thesis to instances in which we ourselves seem most clearly to hear the voice of conscience. We should maintain with the most absolute certainty that we feel not the slightest temptation to violate any of these prohibitions—the commandment to 'do no murder', for instance—and that we feel nothing but horror at the notion of violating them.

If, however, we were to admit the claims thus asserted by our

---

[1] [It is to be remarked that Freud's views on the origin and nature both of conscience and of anxiety were greatly modified in his later writings. For these later views see Lectures 31 and 32 in his *New Introductory Lectures* (1933).]

conscience, it would follow, on the one hand, that these prohibitions would be superfluous—both taboo and our own moral prohibitions—and, on the other hand, the fact of conscience would remain unexplained and no place would be left for the relations between conscience, taboo and neurosis. In other words, we should be back in the state of knowledge we were in before we approached the problem from the psycho-analytic angle.

Suppose, on the other hand, that we were to take into account the finding arrived at by psycho-analysis from the dreams of normal people, to the effect that we ourselves are subject, more strongly and more often than we suspect, to a temptation to kill someone and that that temptation produces psychical effects even though it remains out of sight of our consciousness. Suppose, again, that we were to recognize the compulsive observances of certain neurotics as being guarantees against an intensified impulse to murder or as being self-punishments on account of it. In that case we should have to attach still greater importance to our thesis that where there is a prohibition there must be an underlying desire. We should have to suppose that the desire to murder is actually present in the unconscious and that neither taboos nor moral prohibitions are psychologically superfluous but that on the contrary they are explained and justified by the existence of an ambivalent attitude towards the impulse to murder.

One of the characteristics of this ambivalent relation which I have repeatedly stressed as fundamental—the fact that the positive current of desire is an unconscious one—opens the way to further considerations and to further possible explanations. Psychical processes in the unconscious are not in every respect identical with those with which our conscious mind is familiar; they enjoy some remarkable liberties that are forbidden to the latter. An unconscious impulse need not have arisen at the point where it makes its appearance; it may arise from some quite other region and have applied originally to quite other persons and connections; it may have reached the place at which it attracts our attention through the mechanism of 'displacement'. Owing, moreover, to the indestructibility and insusceptibility to correction which are attributes of unconscious processes, it may have survived from very early times to which it was appropriate into later times and circumstances in which its manifestations are bound to seem strange. These are no more than hints, but if they were attentively developed their importance for our understanding of the growth of civilization would become apparent.

Before I conclude this discussion, a further point must not be overlooked which will pave the way for later inquiries. In maintaining the essential similarity between taboo prohibitions and moral prohibitions, I have not sought to dispute the fact that there must be a psychological difference between them. The only possible reason why the prohibitions no longer take the form of taboos must be some change in the circumstances governing the ambivalence underlying them.

In our analytical examination of the problems of taboo we have hitherto allowed ourselves to be led by the points of agreement that we have been able to show between it and obsessional neurosis. But after all taboo is not a neurosis but a social institution. We are therefore faced with the task of explaining what difference there is in principle between a neurosis and a cultural creation such as taboo.

Once again I will take a single fact as my starting-point. It is feared among primitive peoples that the violation of a taboo will be followed by a punishment, as a rule by some serious illness or by death. The punishment threatens to fall on whoever was responsible for violating the taboo. In obsessional neuroses the case is different. What the patient fears if he performs some forbidden action is that a punishment will fall not on himself but on someone else. This person's identity is as a rule left unstated, but can usually be shown without difficulty by analysis to be one of those closest and most dear to the patient. Here, then, the neurotic seems to be behaving altruistically and the primitive man egoistically. Only if the violation of a taboo is not automatically avenged upon the wrong-doer does a collective feeling arise among savages that they are all threatened by the outrage; and they thereupon hasten to carry out the omitted punishment themselves. There is no difficulty in explaining the mechanism of this solidarity. What is in question is fear of an infectious example, of the temptation to imitate—that is, of the contagious character of taboo. If one person succeeds in gratifying the repressed desire, the same desire is bound to be kindled in all the other members of the community. In order to keep the temptation down, the envied transgressor must be deprived of the fruit of his enterprise; and the punishment will not infrequently give those who carry it out an opportunity of committing the same outrage under colour of an act of expiation. This is indeed one of the foundations of the human penal system and it is based, no doubt correctly, on the assumption that the prohibited impulses are present alike in the criminal and in the avenging community. In this, psycho-analysis is no more than confirming the habitual pronouncement of the pious: we are all miserable sinners.

How, then, are we to account for the unexpected nobility of mind of the neurotic, who fears nothing on his own account but everything for someone he loves? Analytical inquiry shows that this attitude is not primary. Originally, that is to say at the beginning of the illness, the threat of punishment applied, as in the case of savages, to the patient himself; he was invariably in fear for his own life; it was not until later that the mortal fear was displaced on to another and a loved person. The process is a little complicated, but we can follow it perfectly. At the root of the prohibition there is invariably a hostile impulse against someone the patient loves—a wish that that person should die. This impulse is repressed by a prohibition and the prohibition is attached to some particular act, which, by displacement, represents, it may be, a hostile act against the loved person. There is a threat of death if this act is performed. But the process goes further, and the original *wish* that the loved person may die is replaced by a *fear* that he may die. So that when the neurosis appears to be so tenderly altruistic, it is merely *compensating* for an underlying contrary attitude of brutal egoism. We may describe as 'social' the emotions which are determined by showing consideration for another person without taking him as a [direct] sexual object. The receding into the background of these social factors may be stressed as a fundamental characteristic of the neurosis, though one which is later disguised by over-compensation.

Taboo and Emotional Ambivalence

I do not propose to linger over the origin of these social impulses and their relation to the other basic human instincts but
shall proceed to illustrate the second main characteristic of the
neurosis by means of another example. In the forms which it
assumes, taboo very closely resembles the neurotic's fear of
touching, his 'touching phobia'. Now, in the case of the neurosis
the prohibition invariably relates to touching of a *sexual* kind,
and psycho-analysis has shown that it is in general true that the
instinctual forces that are diverted and displaced in neuroses
have a sexual origin. In the case of taboo the prohibited touching is obviously not to be understood in an exclusively sexual
sense but in the more general sense of attacking, of getting control, and of asserting oneself. If there is a prohibition against
touching a chief or anything that has been in contact with him,
this means that an inhibition is to be laid on the same impulse
which expresses itself on other occasions in keeping a suspicious
watch upon the chief or even in ill-treating him physically before his coronation. (See above [p. 49].) Thus the fact which is
characteristic of the neurosis is the preponderance of the sexual
over the social instinctual elements.[1] The social instincts, however, are themselves derived from a combination of egoistic and
erotic components into wholes of a special kind.

This single comparison between taboo and obsessional neurosis is enough to enable us to gather the nature of the relation
between the different forms of neurosis and cultural institutions,
and to see how it is that the study of the psychology of the neuroses is important for an understanding of the growth of civilization.

The neuroses exhibit on the one hand striking and far-reaching points of agreement with those great social institutions, art,
religion and philosophy. But on the other hand they seem like
distortions of them. It might be maintained that a case of hys-
teria is a caricature of a work of art, that an obsessional neurosis
is a caricature of a religion and that a paranoic delusion is a
caricature of a philosophical system. The divergence resolves
itself ultimately into the fact that the neuroses are social structures; they endeavour to achieve by private means what is
effected in society by collective effort. If we analyse the in-

[1] [This sentence is in spaced type in the original.]

73

stincts at work in the neuroses, we find that the determining influence in them is exercised by instinctual forces of sexual origin; the corresponding cultural formations, on the other hand, are based upon social instincts, originating from the combination of egoistic and erotic elements. Sexual needs are not capable of uniting men in the same way as are the demands of self-preservation. Sexual satisfaction is essentially the private affair of each individual.

The asocial nature of neuroses has its genetic origin in their most fundamental purpose, which is to take flight from an unsatisfying reality into a more pleasurable world of phantasy. The real world, which is avoided in this way by neurotics, is under the sway of human society and of the institutions collectively created by it. To turn away from reality is at the same time to withdraw from the community of man.

III

Animism, Magic and the Omnipotence of Thoughts

(1)

WRITINGS that seek to apply the findings of psycho-analysis to topics in the field of the mental sciences have the inevitable defect of offering too little to readers of both classes. Such writings can only be in the nature of an instigation: they put before the specialist certain suggestions for him to take into account in his own work. This defect is bound to be extremely evident in an essay which will attempt to deal with the immense domain of what is known as '*animism*'.[1]

Animism is, in its narrower sense, the doctrine of souls, and, in its wider sense, the doctrine of spiritual beings in general. The term 'animatism' has also been used to denote the theory of the living character of what appear to us to be inanimate objects [see below, p. 91], and the terms 'animalism' and 'manism' occur as well in this connection. The word 'animism', originally used to describe a particular philosophical system, seems to have been given its present meaning by Tylor.[2]

What led to the introduction of these terms was a realization of the highly remarkable view of nature and the universe adopted by the primitive races of whom we have knowledge,

---

[1] The necessity for a concise treatment of the material involves the omission of any elaborate bibliography. Instead, I will merely refer to the standard works of Herbert Spencer, J. G. Frazer, Andrew Lang, E. B. Tylor and Wilhelm Wundt, from which all that I have to say about animism and magic is derived. My own contribution is visible only in my selection both of material and of opinions.

[2] Cf. Tylor (1891, **1**, 425), Wundt (1906 [142 f. and] 173) [and Marett (1900, 171)].

whether in past history or at the present time. They people the world with innumerable spiritual beings both benevolent and malignant; and these spirits and demons they regard as the causes of natural phenomena and they believe that not only animals and plants but all the inanimate objects in the world are animated by them. A third, and perhaps the most important, article of this primitive 'philosophy of nature'[1] strikes us as less strange, since, while we have retained only a very limited belief in the existence of spirits and explain natural phenomena by the agency of impersonal physical forces, we ourselves are not very far removed from this third belief. For primitive peoples believe that human individuals are inhabited by similar spirits. These souls which live in human beings can leave their habitations and migrate into other human beings; they are the vehicle of mental activities and are to a certain extent independent of their bodies. Originally souls were pictured as very similar to persons and only in the course of a long development have they lost their material characteristics and become to a high degree 'spiritualized'.[2]

Most authorities incline to the view that these ideas of a soul are the original nucleus of the animistic system, that spirits are only souls that have made themselves independent, and that the souls of animals, plants and objects were constructed on the analogy of human souls.

How did primitive men arrive at the peculiar dualistic views on which the animistic system is based? It is supposed that they did so by observing the phenomena of sleep (including dreams) and of death which so much resembles it, and by attempting to explain those states, which are of such close concern to everyone. The chief starting-point of this theorizing must have been the problem of death. What primitive man regarded as the natural thing was the indefinite prolongation of life—immortality. The idea of death was only accepted late, and with hesitancy. Even for us it is lacking in content and has no clear connotation. There have been very lively but inconclusive discussions upon the part that may have been played in the formation of the basic doctrines of animism by such other observed or ex-

[1] ['*Naturphilosophie*', the pantheistic philosophy of Schelling.]
[2] Wundt (1906), Chapter IV, 'Die Seelenvorstellungen'.

perienced facts as dream-pictures, shadows, mirror images, and so on.[1]

It has been regarded as perfectly natural and not in the least puzzling that primitive man should have reacted to the phenomena which aroused his speculations by forming the idea of the soul and then of extending it to objects in the external world. In discussing the fact that the same animistic ideas have emerged among the most various races and at every period, Wundt (1906, 154) declares that 'they are the necessary psychological product of a mythopœic consciousness . . . and in this sense, therefore, primitive animism must be regarded as the spiritual expression of the natural state of man, so far as it is accessible to our observation'. The justification for attributing life to inanimate objects was already stated by Hume in his *Natural History of Religion* [Section III]: 'There is an universal tendency among mankind to conceive all beings like themselves, and to transfer to every object those qualities with which they are familiarly acquainted, and of which they are intimately conscious.'[2]

Animism is a system of thought. It does not merely give an explanation of a particular phenomenon, but allows us to grasp the whole universe as a single unity from a single point of view. The human race, if we are to follow the authorities, have in the course of ages developed three such systems of thought—three great pictures of the universe: animistic (or mythological), religious and scientific. Of these, animism, the first to be created, is perhaps the one which is most consistent and exhaustive and which gives a truly complete explanation of the nature of the universe. This first human *Weltanschauung* is a *psychological* theory. It would go beyond our present purpose to show how much of it still persists in modern life, either in the debased form of superstition or as the living basis of our speech, our beliefs and our philosophies.

With these three stages in mind, it may be said that animism itself is not yet a religion but contains the foundations on which religions are later built. It is obvious, too, that myths are based

---

[1] Cf. Wundt [loc. cit.], Herbert Spencer [1893, Part I], as well as the general articles in the *Encyclopaedia Britannica* (1910–11) on 'Animism', 'Mythology', etc.

[2] Quoted by Tylor (1891, **1**, 477).

on animistic premises, though the details of the relation between myths and animism seem to be unexplained in some
essential respects.

(2)

Our psycho-analytic approach to the subject, however, is
from another side. It is not to be supposed that men were inspired to create their first system of the universe by pure specu-
lative curiosity. The practical need for controlling the world
around them must have played its part. So we are not surprised
to learn that, hand in hand with the animistic system, there
went a body of instructions upon how to obtain mastery over
men, beasts and things—or rather, over their spirits. These instructions go by the names of 'sorcery' and 'magic'.[1] Reinach
(1905–12, **2**, xv) describes them as the 'strategy of animism'; I
should prefer, following Hubert and Mauss (1904 [142 ff.]), to
regard them as its technique.

Can the concepts of sorcery and magic be distinguished? Perhaps—if we are prepared to show a somewhat arbitrary disregard for the fluctuations of linguistic usage. Sorcery, then, is
essentially the art of influencing spirits by treating them in the
same way as one would treat men in like circumstances: appeas-
ing them, making amends to them, propitiating them, intimi-
dating them, robbing them of their power, subduing them to
one's will—by the same methods that have proved effective
with living men. Magic, on the other hand, is something different: fundamentally, it disregards spirits and makes use of special
procedures and not of everyday psychological methods. It is
easy to guess that magic is the earlier and more important
branch of animistic technique; for magical methods can, among
others, be used in dealing with spirits,[2] and magic can be applied
as well in cases where, as it seems to us, the process of spiritualiz-
ing Nature has not yet been carried out.

Magic has to serve the most varied purposes—it must subject
natural phenomena to the will of man, it must protect the indi-

---

[1] ['*Zauberei*' and '*Magie*' in the original.]

[2] If a spirit is scared away by making a noise and shouting, the action
is one purely of sorcery; if compulsion is applied to it by getting hold of
its name, magic has been used against it.

vidual from his enemies and from dangers and it must give him power to injure his enemies. But the principle on the presumption of which magical action is based—or, more properly, the principle of magic—is so striking that none of the authorities has failed to recognize it. Tylor [1891, 1, 116], if we leave on one side an accompanying moral judgment, states it in its most succinct form as mistaking an ideal connection for a real one. I will illustrate this feature from two groups of magical acts.

One of the most widespread magical procedures for injuring an enemy is by making an effigy of him from any convenient material. Whether the effigy resembles him is of little account: any object can be 'made into' an effigy of him. Whatever is then done to the effigy, the same thing happens to the detested original; whatever part of the former's body is damaged, the same part of the latter's becomes diseased. The same magical technique may be employed, not only for purposes of private enmity, but also for pious ends and for giving help to gods against malignant demons. I will quote from Frazer (1911a, 1, 67): 'Every night when the sun-god Ra sank down to his home in the glowing west he was assailed by hosts of demons under the leadership of the arch-fiend Apepi. All night long he fought them, and sometimes by day the powers of darkness sent up clouds even into the blue Egyptian sky to obscure his light and weaken his power. To aid the sun-god in this daily struggle, a ceremony was daily performed in his temple at Thebes. A figure of his foe Apepi, represented as a crocodile with a hideous face or a serpent with many coils, was made of wax, and on it the demon's name was written in green ink. Wrapt in a papyrus case, on which another likeness of Apepi had been drawn in green ink, the figure was then tied up with black hair, spat upon, hacked with a stone knife, and cast on the ground. There the priest trod on it with his left foot again and again, and then burnt it in a fire made of a certain plant or grass. When Apepi himself had thus been effectually disposed of, waxen effigies of each of his principal demons, and of their fathers, mothers and children, were made and burnt in the same way. The service, accompanied by the recitation of certain prescribed spells, was repeated not merely morning, noon and night, but whenever a storm was raging, or heavy rain had set in, or black clouds were stealing across the sky to hide the sun's bright disc. The fiends of darkness, clouds, and rain felt the injuries inflicted on their images as if they had been done to themselves; they passed away, at least for a time, and the beneficent sun-god shone out triumphant once more.'[1]

From the vast number of magical acts having a similar basis I will only draw attention to two more, which have played a large part among primitive peoples of every age and which persist to some degree in the myths and cults of higher stages of civilization—that is, rituals for producing rain and fertility. Rain is produced magically by imitating it or the clouds and storms which give rise to it, by 'playing at rain', one might almost say. In Japan, for instance, 'a party of Ainos will scatter water by means of sieves, while others will take a porringer, fit it up with sails and oars as if it were a boat, and then push or draw it about the village and gardens'.[2] In the same way, the fertility of the earth is magically promoted by a dramatic representation of human intercourse. Thus, to take one from a countless number of instances, 'in some parts of Java, at the season when the bloom will soon be on the rice, the husbandman and his wife visit their fields by night and there engage in sexual intercourse' to encourage the fertility of the rice by their example.[3] There is a dread, however, that prohibited, incestuous sexual relations may cause a failure of the crops and make the earth sterile.[4]

Certain negative observances, that is, magical precautions, must be included in this first group. 'When a Dyak village has turned out to hunt wild pigs in the jungle, the people who stay at home may not touch oil or water with their hands during the absence of their friends; for if they did so, the hunters would all be "butter-fingered" and the prey would slip through their

[1] It seems probable that the biblical prohibition against making an image of any living thing originated, not from any objection to the plastic arts, but from a desire to deprive magic (which was abominated by the Hebrew religion) of one of its tools. Cf. Frazer (1911a, 1, 87 n.).
[2] [Frazer (1911a, 1, 251), quoting Batchelor (1901, 333).]
[3] Frazer (1911a, 2, 98) [quoting Wilken (1884, 958)].
[4] An echo of this is to be found in the *Œdipus Rex* of Sophocles [e.g. in the prologue and first Chorus].

hands.'¹ Or again, 'while a Gilyak hunter is pursuing game in the forest, his children at home are forbidden to make drawings on wood or on sand; for they fear that if the children did so, the paths in the forest would become as perplexed as the lines in the drawings, so that the hunter might lose his way and never return.'²

In these last, as in so many other instances of the workings of magic, the element of distance is disregarded; in other words, telepathy is taken for granted. We shall find no difficulty, therefore, in understanding this characteristic of magic.

There can be no doubt what is to be regarded as the operative factor in all these examples. It is the *similarity* between the act performed and the result expected. For this reason Frazer describes this sort of magic as 'imitative' or 'homœopathic'. If I wish it to rain, I have only to do something that looks like rain or is reminiscent of rain. At a later stage of civilization, instead of this rain-magic, processions will be made to a temple and prayers for rain will be addressed to the deity living in it. Finally, this religious technique will in its turn be given up and attempts will be made to produce effects in the atmosphere which will lead to rain.

In a second group of magical acts the principle of similarity plays no part, and its place is taken by another one, the nature of which will at once become clear from the following examples.

There is another procedure by which an enemy can be injured. One gets possession of some of his hair or nails or other waste products or even a piece of his clothing, and treats them in some hostile way. It is then exactly as though one had got possession of the man himself; and he himself experiences whatever it is that has been done to the objects that originated from him. In the view of primitive man, one of the most important parts of a person is his name. So that if one knows the name of a man or of a spirit, one has obtained a certain amount of power over the owner of the name. This is the origin of the remarkable precautions and restrictions in the use of names which we have already touched upon in the essay on taboo. (See p. 54 ff.) In

¹ Frazer (1911*a*, **1**, 120) [quoting Roth (1896, **1**, 430)].
² Frazer (1911*a*, **1**, 122) [quoting Labbé (1903, 268)].

these examples the place of similarity is evidently taken by affinity.

The higher motives for cannibalism among primitive races have a similar origin. By incorporating parts of a person's body through the act of eating, one at the same time acquires the qualities possessed by him. This leads in certain circumstances to precautions and restrictions in regard to diet. A woman who is with child will avoid eating the flesh of certain animals for fear that any undesirable qualities they may have (cowardice, for instance) might be passed over to the child that is nourished by her. The magical power is not affected even if the connection between the two objects has already been severed or even if the contact occurred only on a single important occasion. For instance, the belief that there is a magical bond between a wound and the weapon which caused it may be traced unaltered for thousands of years. If a Melanesian can obtain possession of the bow which caused his wound, he will keep it carefully in a cool place so as to reduce the inflammation of the wound. But if the bow was left in the enemy's possession, it will undoubtedly be hung up close to the fire so that the wound may become thoroughly hot and inflamed.[1] Pliny (in his *Natural History*, Book xxviii [Chapter 7]) tells us that 'if you have wounded a man and are sorry for it, you have only to spit on the hand that gave the wound, and the pain of the sufferer will be instantly alleviated'. [Frazer, loc. cit.] So, too, Francis Bacon (in his *Sylva Sylvarum* [X, § 998]) mentions that 'it is constantly received and avouched that the anointing of the weapon that maketh the wound will heal the wound itself'. English country people are said even to-day to follow this prescription, and if they cut themselves with a scythe carefully keep the instrument clean, to prevent the wound from festering. 'At Norwich in June 1902 a woman named Matilda Henry accidentally ran a nail into her foot. Without examining the wound, or even removing her stocking, she caused her daughter to grease the nail, saying that if this were done no harm would come of the hurt. A few days afterwards she died of lockjaw'—as a result of this displaced antisepsis. (Frazer, ibid., 203.)

The last group of instances exemplify what Frazer distin-

[1] [Frazer (1911a, 1, 201), quoting Codrington (1891, 310).]

82

guishes from 'imitative' magic under the name of 'contagious' magic. What is believed to be their effective principle is no longer similarity but spacial connection, contiguity, or at least *imagined* contiguity—the recollection of it. Since, however, similarity and contiguity are the two essential principles of processes of association, it appears that the true explanation of all the folly of magical observances is the domination of the association of ideas. The aptness of Tylor's description of magic which I have already quoted [p. 79] now becomes evident: mistaking an ideal connection for a real one. Frazer (1911a, 1, 420) has put it almost in the same words: 'Men mistook the order of their ideas for the order of nature, and hence imagined that the control which they have, or seem to have, over their thoughts, permitted them to exercise a corresponding control over things.'

We shall at first be surprised to learn that this illuminating explanation of magic has been rejected by some writers as unsatisfactory (e.g. Thomas, 1910–11a). On reflection, however, it will be seen that the criticism is justified. The associative theory of magic merely explains the paths along which magic proceeds; it does not explain its true essence, namely the misunderstanding which leads it to replace the laws of nature by psychological ones. Some dynamic factor is evidently missing. But whereas the critics of Frazer's theory have gone astray in their search for it, it will be easy to arrive at a satisfactory explanation of magic merely by carrying the associative theory further and deeper.

Let us consider first the simpler and more important case of imitative magic. According to Frazer (1911a, 1, 54) it can be practised by itself, whereas contagious magic as a rule presupposes the other. It is easy to perceive the motives which lead men to practise magic: they are human wishes. All we need to suppose is that primitive man had an immense belief in the power of his wishes. The basic reason why what he sets about by magical means comes to pass is, after all, simply that he wills it. To begin with, therefore, the emphasis is only upon his wish.

Children are in an analogous psychical situation, though their motor efficiency is still undeveloped. I have elsewhere (1911a) put forward the hypothesis that, to begin with, they satisfy their wishes in an hallucinatory manner, that is, they create a satisfying situation by means of centrifugal excitations of their sense organs. An adult primitive man has an alternative method open to him. His wishes are accompanied by a motor impulse, the will, which is later destined to alter the whole face of the earth in order to satisfy his wishes. This motor impulse is at first employed to give a representation of the satisfying situation in such a way that it becomes possible to experience the satisfaction by means of what might be described as motor hallucinations. This kind of representation of a satisfied wish is quite comparable to children's play, which succeeds their earlier purely sensory technique of satisfaction. If children and primitive men find play and imitative representation enough for them, that is not a sign of their being unassuming in our sense or of their resignedly accepting their actual impotence. It is the easily understandable result of the paramount virtue they ascribe to their wishes, of the will that is associated with those wishes and of the methods by which those wishes operate. As time goes on, the psychological accent shifts from the *motives* for the magical act on to the *measures* by which it is carried out—that is, on to the act itself. (It would perhaps be more correct to say that it is only these measures that reveal to the subject the excessive valuation which he attaches to his psychical acts.) It thus comes to appear as though it is the magical act itself which, owing to its similarity with the desired result, alone determines the occurrence of that result. There is no opportunity, at the stage of animistic thinking, for showing any objective evidence of the true state of affairs. But a possibility of doing so *does* arrive at a later time, when, though all of these procedures are still being carried out, the psychical phenomenon of doubt has begun to emerge as an expression of a tendency to repression. At that point, men will be ready to admit that conjuring up spirits has no result unless it is accompanied by faith, and that the magical power of prayer fails if there is no piety at work behind it.[1]

The fact that it has been possible to construct a system of contagious magic on associations of contiguity shows that the im-

---

[1] Cf. the King in *Hamlet* (III. 3):
    'My words fly up, my thoughts remain below:
    Words without thoughts never to heaven go.'

portance attached to wishes and to the will has been extended from them on to all those psychical acts which are subject to the will. A general over-valuation has thus come about of all mental processes—an attitude towards the world, that is, which, in view of our knowledge of the relation between reality and thought, cannot fail to strike *us* as an over-valuation of the latter. Things become less important than ideas of things: whatever is done to the latter will inevitably also occur to the former. Relations which hold between the ideas of things are assumed to hold equally between the things themselves. Since distance is of no importance in thinking—since what lies furthest apart both in time and space can without difficulty be comprehended in a single act of consciousness—so, too, the world of magic has a telepathic disregard for spacial distance and treats past situations as though they were present. In the animistic epoch the reflection of the internal world is bound to blot out the other picture of the world—the one which *we* seem to perceive.

It is further to be noticed that the two principles of association —similarity and contiguity—are both included in the more comprehensive concept of 'contact'. Association by contiguity is contact in the literal sense; association by similarity is contact in the metaphorical sense. The use of the same word for the two kinds of relation is no doubt accounted for by some identity in the psychical processes concerned which we have not yet grasped. We have here the same range of meaning of the idea of 'contact' as we found in our analysis of taboo.[1]

By way of summary, then, it may be said that the principle governing magic, the technique of the animistic mode of thinking, is the principle of the 'omnipotence of thoughts'.

(3)

I have adopted the term 'omnipotence of thoughts' from a highly intelligent man who suffered from obsessional ideas and who, after having been set right by psycho-analytical treatment, was able to give evidence of his efficiency and good sense. (Cf. Freud, 1909*b*.) He had coined the phrase as an explanation of all the strange and uncanny events by which he, like others

[1] Cf. the second essay in this volume [p. 27].

G   85

afflicted with the same illness, seemed to be pursued. If he thought of someone, he would be sure to meet that very person immediately afterwards, as though by magic. If he suddenly asked after the health of an acquaintance whom he had not seen for a long time, he would hear that he had just died, so that it would look as though a telepathic message had arrived from him. If, without any really serious intention, he swore at some stranger, he might be sure that the man would die soon afterwards, so that he would feel responsible for his death. In the course of the treatment he himself was able to tell me how the deceptive appearance arose in most of these cases, and by what contrivances he himself had helped to strengthen his own superstitious beliefs. All obsessional neurotics are superstitious in this way, usually against their better judgment.[1]

It is in obsessional neuroses that the survival of the omnipotence of thoughts is most clearly visible and that the consequences of this primitive mode of thinking come closest to consciousness. But we must not be misled into supposing that it is a distinguishing feature of this particular neurosis, for analytic investigation reveals the same thing in the other neuroses as well. In all of them what determines the formation of symptoms is the reality not of experience but of thought. Neurotics live in a world apart, where, as I have said elsewhere [1911a, English translation, 20], only 'neurotic currency' is legal tender; that is to say, they are only affected by what is thought with intensity and pictured with emotion, whereas agreement with external reality is a matter of no importance. What hysterics repeat in their attacks and fix by means of their symptoms are experiences which have occurred in that form only in their imagination— though it is true that in the last resort those imagined experiences go back to actual events or are based upon them. To attribute the neurotic sense of guilt to real misdeeds would show an equal misunderstanding. An obsessional neurotic may be weighed down by a sense of guilt that would be appropriate in a

---

[1] We appear to attribute an 'uncanny' quality to impressions that seek to confirm the omnipotence of thoughts and the animistic mode of thinking in general, after we have reached a stage at which, in our *judgment*, we have abandoned such beliefs. [Cf. Freud's subsequent paper on 'The Uncanny' (1919).]

mass-murderer, while in fact, from his childhood onwards, he has behaved to his fellow-men as the most considerate and scrupulous member of society. Nevertheless, his sense of guilt has a justification: it is founded on the intense and frequent death-wishes against his fellows which are unconsciously at work in him. It has a justification if what we take into account are unconscious thoughts and not intentional deeds. Thus the omnipotence of thoughts, the over-valuation of mental processes as compared with reality, is seen to have unrestricted play in the emotional life of neurotic patients and in everything that derives from it. If one of them undergoes psycho-analytic treatment, which makes what is unconscious in him conscious, he will be unable to believe that thoughts are free and will constantly be afraid of expressing evil wishes, as though their expression would lead inevitably to their fulfilment. This behaviour, as well as the superstitions which he practises in ordinary life, reveals his resemblance to the savages who believe they can alter the external world by mere thinking.

The primary obsessive acts of these neurotics are of an entirely magical character. If they are not charms, they are at all events counter-charms, designed to ward off the expectations of disaster with which the neurosis usually starts. Whenever I have succeeded in penetrating the mystery, I have found that the expected disaster was death. Schopenhauer has said that the problem of death stands at the outset of every philosophy; and we have already seen [p. 65] that the origin of the belief in souls and in demons, which is the essence of animism, goes back to the impression which is made upon men by death. It is difficult to judge whether the obsessive or protective acts performed by obsessional neurotics follow the law of similarity (or, as the case may be, of contrast); for as a rule, owing to the prevailing conditions of the neurosis, they have been distorted by being displaced on to some detail, on to some action which is in itself of the greatest triviality.[1] The protective formulas of obsessional neuroses, too, have their counterpart in the formulas of magic. It is possible, however, to describe the course of development of obsessive acts: we can show how they begin by being as remote

[1] A further motive for such displacement on to a trivial action will appear in what follows.

as possible from anything sexual—magical defences against evil wishes—and how they end by being substitutes for the forbidden sexual act and the closest possible imitations of it.

If we are prepared to accept the account given above of the evolution of human views of the universe—an animistic phase followed by a religious phase and this in turn by a scientific one —it will not be difficult to follow the vicissitudes of the 'omnipotence of thoughts' through these different phases. At the animistic stage men ascribe omnipotence to *themselves*. At the religious stage they transfer it to the gods but do not seriously abandon it themselves, for they reserve the power of influencing the gods in a variety of ways according to their wishes. The scientific view of the universe no longer affords any room for human omnipotence; men have acknowledged their smallness and submitted resignedly to death and to the other necessities of nature. None the less some of the primitive belief in omnipotence still survives in men's faith in the power of the human mind, taking account, as it does, of the laws of reality.

If we trace back the development of libidinal trends as we find them in the individual from their adult forms to the first beginnings in childhood, an important distinction emerges, which I have described in my *Three Essays on the Theory of Sexuality* (1905*a*). Manifestations of the sexual instincts can be observed from the very first, but to begin with they are not yet directed towards any external object. The separate instinctual components of sexuality work independently of one another to obtain pleasure and find satisfaction in the subject's own body. This stage is known as that of auto-erotism and it is succeeded by one in which an object is chosen.

Further study has shown that it is expedient and indeed indispensable to insert a third stage between these two, or, putting it in another way, to divide the first stage, that of auto-erotism, into two. At this intermediate stage, the importance of which is being made more and more evident by research, the hitherto isolated sexual instincts have already come together into a single whole and have also found an object. But this object is not an external one, extraneous to the subject, but it is his own ego, which has been constituted at about this same time. Bearing in mind pathological fixations of this new stage, which become observable later, we have given it the name of 'narcissism'. The subject behaves as though he were in love with himself; his egoistic instincts and his libidinal wishes are not yet separable under our analysis.

Although we are not yet in a position to describe with sufficient accuracy the characteristics of this narcissistic stage, at which the hitherto dissociated sexual instincts come together into a single unity and cathect[1] the ego as an object, we suspect already that this narcissistic organization is never wholly abandoned. A human being remains to some extent narcissistic even after he has found external objects for his libido. The cathexes of objects which he effects are as it were emanations of the libido that still remains in his ego and can be drawn back into it once more. The state of being in love, which is psychologically so remarkable and is the normal prototype of the psychoses, shows these emanations at their maximum compared to the level of self-love.

Primitive men and neurotics, as we have seen, attach a high valuation—in our eyes an *over*-valuation—to psychical acts. This attitude may plausibly be brought into relation with narcissism and regarded as an essential component of it. It may be said that in primitive men the process of thinking is still to a great extent sexualized. This is the origin of their belief in the omnipotence of thoughts, their unshakable confidence in the possibility of controlling the world and their inaccessibility to the experiences, so easily obtainable, which could teach them man's true position in the universe. As regards neurotics, we find that on the one hand a considerable part of this primitive attitude has survived in their constitution, and on the other hand that the sexual repression that has occurred in them has brought about a further sexualization of their thinking processes. The psychological results must be the same in both cases, whether the libidinal hypercathexis of thinking is an original one or has

---

[1] [The words 'cathexis' and 'to cathect' are used as renderings of the German *'Besetzung'* and *'besetzen'*. They are the terms with which Freud expresses the idea of psychical energy being lodged in or attaching itself to mental structures or processes, somewhat on the analogy of an electric charge.]

been produced by regression: intellectual narcissism and the omnipotence of thoughts.[1]

If we may regard the existence among primitive races of the omnipotence of thoughts as evidence in favour of narcissism, we are encouraged to attempt a comparison between the phases in the development of men's view of the universe and the stages of an individual's libidinal development. The animistic phase would correspond to narcissism both chronologically and in its content; the religious phase would correspond to the stage of object-choice of which the characteristic is a child's attachment to his parents; while the scientific phase would have an exact counterpart in the stage at which an individual has reached maturity, has renounced the pleasure principle, adjusted himself to reality and turned to the external world for the object of his desires.[2]

In only a single field of our civilization has the omnipotence of thoughts been retained, and that is in the field of art. Only in art does it still happen that a man who is consumed by desires performs something resembling the accomplishment of those desires and that what he does in play produces emotional effects —thanks to artistic illusion—just as though it were something real. People speak with justice of the 'magic of art' and compare artists to magicians. But the comparison is perhaps more significant than it claims to be. There can be no doubt that art did not begin as art for art's sake. It worked originally in the service of impulses which are for the most part extinct to-day. And among them we may suspect the presence of many magical purposes.[3]

[1] 'It is almost an axiom with writers on this subject, that a sort o Solipsism, or Berkleianism (as Professor Sully terms it as he finds it in the Child), operates in the savage to make him refuse to recognize death as a fact.' (Marett, 1900, 178.)

[2] I will only briefly allude here to the fact that the original narcissism of children has a decisive influence upon our view of the development of their character and excludes the possibility of their having any primary sense of inferiority.

[3] Cf. Reinach, 'L'art et la magie' (1905–12, 1, 125–36). In Reinach's opinion the primitive artists who left behind the carvings and paintings of animals in the French caves, did not desire to 'please' but to 'evoke' or conjure up. He thus explains why it is that these pictures are situated in the darkest and most inaccessible parts of the caves and that dangerous

(4)

Thus the first picture which man formed of the world—animism—was a psychological one. It needed no scientific basis as yet, since science only begins after it has been realized that the world is unknown and that means must therefore be sought for getting to know it. Animism came to primitive man naturally and as a matter of course. He knew what things were like in the world, namely just as he felt himself to be. We are thus prepared to find that primitive man transposed the structural conditions of his own mind[1] into the external world; and we may attempt to reverse the process and put back into the human mind what animism teaches as to the nature of things.

The technique of animism, magic, reveals in the clearest and most unmistakable way an intention to impose the laws governing mental life upon real things; in this, spirits need not as yet play any part, though spirits may be taken as objects of magical treatment. Thus the assumptions of magic are more fundamental and older than the doctrine of spirits, which forms the kernel of animism. Our psycho-analytic point of view coincides here with a theory put forward by R. R. Marett (1900), who postulates a pre-animistic stage before animism, the character of which is best indicated by the term 'animatism', the doctrine of the universality of life. Experience has little light to throw on pre-animism, since no race has yet been discovered which is without the concept of spirits. (Cf. Wundt, 1906, 171 ff.)

Whereas magic still reserves omnipotence solely for thoughts,

beasts of prey do not appear among them. 'Les modernes parlent souvent, par hyperbole, de la magie du pinceau ou du ciseau d'un grand artiste et, en général, de la magie de l'art. Entendu au sens propre, qui est celui d'une contrainte mystique exercée par la volonté de l'homme sur d'autres volontés ou sur les choses, cette expression n'est plus admissible; mais nous avons vu qu'elle était autrefois rigoureusement vraie, du moins dans l'opinion des artistes.' (Ibid., 136.) ['In modern times people often speak metaphorically of the magic of a great artist's brush or chisel, or more generally of the magic of art. This expression is no longer permissible in its proper sense of a mystical force brought to bear by the human will upon other wills or upon objects; but, as we have seen, there was a time when it was literally true—at least in the artists' opinion.']

[1] Which he was aware of by what is known as endopsychic perception.

animism hands some of it over to spirits and so prepares the way for the construction of a religion. What, we may ask, can have induced a primitive man to make this first act of renunciation? It can scarcely have been a recognition of the falseness of his premises, for he continued to practise the magical technique.

Spirits and demons, as I have shown in the last essay, are only projections of man's own emotional impulses.[1] He turns his emotional cathexes into persons, he peoples the world with them and meets his internal mental processes again outside himself—in just the same way as that intelligent paranoiac, Schreber, found a reflection of the attachments and detachments of his libido in the vicissitudes of his confabulated 'rays of God'.[2]

I propose to avoid (as I have already done elsewhere[3]) entering into the general problem of the origin of the tendency to project mental processes into the outside. It is, however, safe to assume that that tendency will be intensified when projection promises to bring with it the advantage of mental relief. Such an advantage may be expected with certainty where a conflict has arisen between different impulses all of which are striving towards omnipotence—for they clearly cannot *all* become omnipotent. The pathological process in paranoia in fact makes use of the mechanism of projection in order to deal with mental conflicts of this kind. The typical case of such a conflict is one between the two members of a pair of opposites—the case of an ambivalent attitude, which we have examined in detail as it appears in someone mourning the death of a loved relative. [Cf. p. 60 ff.] This kind of case must seem particularly likely to provide a motive for the creation of projections. Here again we are in agreement with the writers who maintain that the first-born spirits were *evil* spirits, and who derive the idea of a soul from the impression made by death upon the survivors. The only difference is that *we* do not lay stress on the *intellectual* problem with which death confronts the living; in our view the force

---

[1] I assume that at this early narcissistic stage cathexes arising from libidinal and from other sources of excitation may still be indistinguishable from one another.

[2] Cf. Schreber (1903) and Freud (1911*b*).

[3] In my paper on Schreber (Freud, 1911*b* [English translation, 452]).

which gives the impetus to research is rather to be attributed to the *emotional* conflict into which the survivors are plunged.

Thus man's first theoretical achievement—the creation of spirits—seems to have arisen from the same source as the first moral restrictions to which he was subjected—the observances of taboo. The fact that they had the same origin need not imply, however, that they arose simultaneously. If the survivors' position in relation to the dead was really what first caused primitive man to reflect, and compelled him to hand over some of his omnipotence to the spirits and to sacrifice some of his freedom of action, then these cultural products would constitute a first acknowledgment of 'Ἀνάγκη [Necessity], which opposes human narcissism. Primitive man would thus be submitting to the supremacy of death with the same gesture with which he seemed to be denying it.

If we may venture to exploit our hypothesis still further, we may inquire which essential part of our psychological structure is reflected and reproduced in the projective creation of souls and spirits. It could scarcely be disputed that the primitive conception of a soul, however much it may differ from the later, purely immaterial soul, is nevertheless intrinsically the same; that is to say, it assumes that both persons and things are of a double nature and that their known attributes and modifications are distributed between their two component portions. This original 'duality', to borrow an expression from Herbert Spencer (1893), is identical with the dualism proclaimed by our current distinction between soul and body and by such ineradicable linguistic expressions of it as the use of phrases like 'beside himself' or 'coming to himself' in relation to fits of rage or fainting (ibid., 144).

When we, no less than primitive man, project something into external reality, what is happening must surely be this: we are recognizing the existence of two states—one in which something is directly given to the senses and to consciousness (that is, is *present* to them), and alongside it another, in which the same thing is *latent* but capable of re-appearing. In short, we are recognizing the co-existence of perception and memory, or, putting it more generally, the existence of *unconscious* mental processes alongside the *conscious* ones.[1] It might be said that in the last analysis the 'spirit' of persons or things comes down to their capacity to be remembered and imagined after perception of them has ceased.

It is not, of course, to be expected that either the primitive or the present-day concept of a 'soul' will be separated from that of the other portion of the personality by the same line of demarcation which our modern science draws between conscious and unconscious mental activity. The animistic soul unites properties from both sides. Its volatile and mobile quality, its power of leaving the body and of taking possession, temporarily or permanently, of another body—these are characteristics which remind us unmistakably of the nature of consciousness. But the way in which it remains concealed behind the manifest personality is reminiscent of the unconscious; immutability and indestructibility are qualities which we no longer attribute to conscious but rather to unconscious processes, and we regard the latter as the true vehicle of mental activity.

I have already said that animism is a system of thought, the first complete theory of the universe, and I shall now go on to draw certain conclusions from the psycho-analytic view of such systems. Every day of our lives our experience is in a position to show us the principal characteristics of a 'system'. We have dreams during the night and we have learnt how to interpret them during the day. Dreams may, without contradicting their nature, appear confused and disconnected. But they may, on the contrary, simulate the orderly impressions of a real experience, they may make one event follow from another and make one portion of their content refer to another. Such a result can be more or less successfully achieved; but it scarcely ever succeeds so completely as to leave no absurdity, no rift in its texture, visible. When we come to submit a dream to interpretation, we find that the erratic and irregular arrangement of its constituent parts is quite unimportant from the point of view of our understanding it. The essential elements in a dream are the

[1] Cf. my short paper, 'A Note on the Unconscious in Psycho-Analysis', first published in the *Proceedings* of the Society for Psychical Research in 1912.

dream-thoughts, and these have meaning, connection and order. But their order is quite other than that remembered by us in the manifest content of the dream. In the latter the connection between the dream-thoughts has been abandoned and may either remain completely lost or be replaced by the new connection exhibited in the manifest content. The elements of the dream, apart from their being condensed, are almost invariably arranged in a new order more or less independent of their earlier arrangement. Finally, it must be added that whatever the original material of the dream-thoughts has been turned into by the dream-activity is then subjected to a further influence. This is what is known as 'secondary revision',[1] and its purpose is evidently to get rid of the disconnectedness and unintelligibility produced by the dream-activity and replace it by a new 'meaning'. But this new meaning, arrived at by secondary revision, is no longer the meaning of the dream-thoughts.[2]

The secondary revision of the product of dream-activity is an admirable example of the nature and pretensions of a system. There is an intellectual function in us which demands unity, connection and intelligibility from any material, whether of perception or thought, that comes within its grasp; and if, as a result of special circumstances, it is unable to establish a true connection, it does not hesitate to fabricate a false one. Systems constructed in this way are known to us not only from dreams, but also from phobias, from obsessive thinking and from delusions. The construction of systems is seen most strikingly in delusional disorders (in paranoia), where it dominates the symptomatic picture; but its occurrence in other forms of neuro-psychosis must not be overlooked. In all these cases it can be shown that a rearrangement of the psychical material has been made with a fresh aim in view; and the rearrangement may often have to be a drastic one if the outcome is to be made to appear intelligible from the point of view of the system. Thus a system is best characterized by the fact that at least two reasons can be discovered for each of its products: a reason based upon the pre-

---

[1] ['*Sekundäre Bearbeitung*.' The usual but misleading English translation of this term is 'secondary elaboration'.]

[2] [Cf. *The Interpretation of Dreams* (1900), English translation, 1932, 451 ff.]

mises of the system (a reason, then, which may be delusional) and a concealed reason, which we must judge to be the truly operative and the real one.

This may be illustrated by an example from a neurosis. In my essay on taboo I mentioned a woman patient of mine whose obsessional prohibitions showed the most perfect agreement with a Maori taboo (p. 28). This woman's neurosis was aimed at her husband and culminated in her defence against an unconscious wish that he should die. Her manifest, systematic phobia, however, related to the mention of death in general, while her husband was entirely excluded from it and was never an object of her conscious solicitude. One day she heard her husband giving instructions that his razors, which had lost their edge, were to be taken to a particular shop to be re-set. Driven by a strange uneasiness, she herself set off for the shop. After reconnoitring the ground, she came back and insisted that her husband should get rid of the razors for good and all, since she had discovered that next door to the shop he had named there was an undertaker's establishment: owing to the plan he had made, she said, the razors had become inextricably involved with thoughts of death. This, then, was the *systematic* reason for her prohibition. We may be quite sure that, even without her discovery of the next-door shop, the patient would have come home with a prohibition against the razors. It would have been enough if she had met a hearse on her way to the shop, or someone dressed in mourning or carrying a funeral wreath. The net of possible determinants for the prohibition was spread wide enough to catch the quarry in any event; it merely depended on her decision whether to draw it together or not. It could be shown that on other occasions she would not put the determinants into operation, and she would explain this by saying it had been 'a better day'. The *real* cause of her prohibition upon the razors was, of course, as it was easy to discover, her repugnance to attaching any pleasurable feeling to the idea that her husband might cut his throat with the newly ground razors.

In just the same way, an inhibition upon movement (an abasia or an agoraphobia) will gradually become more complete and more detailed, when once that system has succeeded in installing itself as a representative of an unconscious wish and of the defence against the wish. Whatever other unconscious phantasies and operative reminiscences may be present in the patient force their way to expression as symptoms along this same path, once it has been opened, and group themselves into an appropriate new arrangement within the framework of the inhibition upon movement. Thus it would be a vain and indeed a foolish task to attempt to understand the complexities and details of the symptoms of (for example) an agoraphobia on the basis of its underlying premises; for the whole consistency and strictness of the combination are merely *apparent*. Just as with the façades of dreams, if we look more attentively we find the most blatant inconsistency and arbitrariness in the structure of symptoms. The real reason for the details of a systematic phobia of this kind lies in concealed determinants, which need have nothing to do with an inhibition upon movement; and that, too, is why these phobias take such various and contradictory shapes in different people.

Let us now return to the animistic system with which we are dealing. The insight we have gained into *other* psychological systems enables us to conclude that with primitive man, too, 'superstition' need not be the only or the real reason for some particular custom or observance and does not excuse us from the duty of searching for its hidden motives. Under the domination of an animistic system it is inevitable that every observance and every activity shall have a systematic basis, which nowadays we describe as 'superstitious'. 'Superstition'—like 'anxiety', 'dreams' and 'demons'—is one of those provisional psychological concepts which have crumbled under the impact of psychoanalytic research. Once we have penetrated behind these constructions, which are like screens erected as defences against correct understanding, we begin to realize that the mental life and cultural level of savages have not hitherto had all the recognition they deserve.

If we take instinctual repression as a measure of the level of civilization that has been reached, we shall have to admit that even under the animistic system advances and developments took place which are unjustly despised on account of their superstitious basis. When we are told that the warriors in a savage tribe practise the greatest continence and cleanliness when

97

they go on the war-path, the explanation is put forward that their motive is 'a fear lest the enemy should obtain the refuse of their persons, and thus be enabled to work their destruction by magic' (Frazer, 1911*b*, 157); and an analogous superstitious reason could be suggested for their continence. None the less the fact remains that they have made an instinctual renunciation; and we can understand the position better if we suppose that the savage warrior submits to these restrictions as a counter-measure because he is on the point of yielding completely to the satisfaction of cruel and hostile impulses which are as a rule prohibited to him. The same is true of the numerous cases of sexual restrictions being imposed on anyone who is engaged on difficult or responsible work (ibid., 200 f.). Though the grounds alleged for these prohibitions may belong to a magical context, yet the fundamental idea of gaining greater strength by renouncing some instinctual satisfaction remains unmistakable; and the hygienic root of the prohibition which lies alongside its magical rationalization must not be overlooked. When the men of a savage tribe go out on an expedition to hunt, to fish, to fight or to gather precious plants, their wives left at home are subjected to many oppressive restrictions, to which the savages themselves ascribe a favourable influence, operating at a distance upon the success of the expedition. But it requires very little penetration to see that this factor which operates at a distance is nothing other than the absent men's longing thoughts of home, and that behind these disguises lies a sound piece of psychological insight that the men will only do their best if they feel completely secure about the women whom they have left behind them unguarded. Sometimes they will even themselves declare, without alleging any magical reasons, that a wife's infidelity in marriage will bring to nothing the efforts of an absent husband engaged on some responsible work.

The countless taboo regulations to which the women in savage communities are subject during menstruation are said to be due to a superstitious horror of blood, and this is no doubt in fact one of their determinants. But it would be wrong to overlook the possibility that in this case the horror of blood also serves æsthetic and hygienic purposes, which are obliged in every case to cloak themselves behind magical motives.

Animism, Magic and the Omnipotence of Thoughts

I am under no illusion that in putting forward these attempted explanations I am laying myself open to the charge of endowing modern savages with a subtlety in their mental activities which exceeds all probability. It seems to me quite possible, however, that the same may be true of our attitude towards the psychology of those races that have remained at the animistic level as is true of our attitude towards the mental life of children, which we adults no longer understand and whose fullness and delicacy of feeling we have in consequence so greatly underestimated.

One further group of taboo observances, which have not hitherto been accounted for, deserve mention, since they admit of an explanation which is familiar to psycho-analysts. Among many savage peoples there is a prohibition against keeping sharp weapons or cutting instruments in a house. Frazer (1911b, 238) quotes a German superstition to the effect that a knife should not be left edge upwards, for fear that God and the angels might be injured on it. May we not recognize in this taboo a premonitory warning against possible 'symptomatic acts' in the execution of which a sharp weapon might be employed by unconscious evil impulses?

IV

The Return of Totemism in Childhood

THERE are no grounds for fearing that psycho-analysis, which first discovered that psychical acts and structures are invariably over-determined,[1] will be tempted to trace the origin of anything so complicated as religion to a single source. If psycho-analysis is compelled—and is, indeed, in duty bound—to lay all the emphasis upon one particular source, that does not mean it is claiming either that that source is the only one or that it occupies first place among the numerous contributory factors. Only when we can synthesize the findings in the different fields of research will it become possible to arrive at the relative importance of the part played in the genesis of religion by the mechanism discussed in these pages. Such a task lies beyond the means as well as beyond the purposes of a psycho-analyst.

(1)

In the first of this series of essays we became acquainted with the concept of totemism. We heard that totemism is a system which takes the place of a religion among certain primitive peoples of Australia, America and Africa, and provides the basis of their social organization. As we have heard, it was a Scotsman, McLennan, who in 1869 first drew general attention to the phenomena of totemism (which had hitherto been regarded as mere curiosities) by giving voice to a suspicion that a large number of customs and usages current in various societies ancient and modern were to be explained as remnants of a totemic age. Since that date science has fully accepted his esti-

[1] [I.e. have two or more simultaneous determinants.]

mate of totemism. Let me quote, as one of the most recent statements on the subject, a passage from Wundt's *Elemente der Völkerpsychologie* (1912, 139): 'In the light of all these facts, the conclusion appears highly probable that at some time totemic culture everywhere paved the way for a more advanced civilization, and, thus, that it represents a transitional stage between the age of primitive men and the era of heroes and gods.' [English translation, 139.]

The purpose of the present essays obliges us to enter more deeply into the nature of totemism. For reasons which will presently become clear I will begin with an account given by Reinach, who, in 1900,[1] sketched out a *'Code du totémisme'* in twelve Articles—a catechism, as it were, of the totemic religion:

(1) Certain animals may neither be killed nor eaten, but individual members of the species are reared by human beings and cared for by them.

(2) An animal which has died an accidental death is mourned over and buried with the same honours as a member of the clan.

(3) In some instances the eating prohibition extends only to one particular part of the animal's body.

(4) When one of the animals which are usually spared has to be killed under the stress of necessity, apologies are offered to it and an attempt is made by means of various artifices and evasions to mitigate the violation of the taboo—that is to say, of the murder.

(5) When the animal is made the victim of a ritual sacrifice, it is solemnly bewailed.

(6) On particular solemn occasions and at religious ceremonies the skins of certain animals are worn. Where totemism is still in force, they are the totem animals.

(7) Clans and individuals adopt the names of animals—viz. of the totem animals.

(8) Many clans make use of representations of animals on their standards and weapons; the men have pictures of animals painted or tattooed on their bodies.

(9) If the totem is a formidable or dangerous animal, it is supposed to spare members of the clan named after it.

[1] Cf. Reinach (1905–12, **1**, 17 ff.).

(10) The totem animal protects and gives warning to members of its clan.

(11) The totem animal foretells the future to the loyal members of its clan and serves them as guide.

(12) The members of the totemic clan often believe that they are related to the totem animal by the bond of a common ancestry.

This catechism of the totemic religion can only be seen at its proper value if we take into account the fact that Reinach has included in it all the indications and traces from which the earlier existence of a totemic system can be inferred. The author's peculiar attitude to the problem is shown by his partial neglect of the essential features of totemism. As we shall see, he has relegated one of the two principal articles of the totemic catechism to the background and entirely overlooked the other.

To obtain a correct picture of the nature of totemism we must turn to another author, who has devoted a four-volume work to the subject, which combines the fullest collection of the relevant observations with the most detailed discussion of the problems they raise. We shall remain indebted to J. G. Frazer, the author of *Totemism and Exogamy* (1910), both for enjoyment and instruction, even if psycho-analytic research may lead to conclusions which differ widely from his.[1]

[1] It may be as well, however, to warn the reader, in advance, of the difficulties with which any statements on the subject have to contend.
In the first place, those who collect the observations are not the same as those who examine and discuss them. The former are travellers and missionaries while the latter are students who may never have set eyes on the objects of their researches. Again, communication with savages is not an easy matter. The observers are not always acquainted with the native language but may be obliged to rely on the help of interpreters or to conduct their inquiries through the medium of pidgin-English. Savages are not communicative on the subject of the most intimate details of their cultural life and they talk openly only to those foreigners who have lived among them for many years. They often give false or misleading information for a great variety of motives. (Cf. Frazer, 1910, **1**, 150 f.) It should not be forgotten that primitive races are not young races but are in fact as old as civilized races. There is no reason to suppose that, for the benefit of our information, they have retained their original ideas and institutions undeveloped and undistorted. On the

The Return of Totemism in Childhood

'A totem', wrote Frazer in his first essay on the subject,[1] 'is a class of material objects which a savage regards with superstitious respect, believing that there exists between him and every member of the class an intimate and altogether special relation. . . . The connection between a man and his totem is mutually beneficent; the totem protects the man, and the man shows his respect for the totem in various ways, by not killing it if it be an animal, and not cutting or gathering it if it be a plant. As distinguished from a fetish, a totem is never an isolated individual, but always a class of objects, generally a species of animals or of plants, more rarely a class of inanimate natural objects, very rarely a class of artificial objects. . . .

'Totems are of at least three kinds: (1) the clan totem, common to a whole clan, and passing by inheritance from generation to generation; (2) the sex totem, common either to all the males or to all the females of a tribe, to the exclusion in either case of the other sex; (3) the individual totem, belonging to a single individual and not passing to his descendants. . . .'

The last two kinds of totem do not compare in significance with the clan totem. Unless we are quite mistaken, they are late developments and of little importance for the essential nature of the totem.

'The clan totem is reverenced by a body of men and women who call themselves by the name of the totem, believe themselves to be of one blood, descendants of a common ancestor, and are bound together by common obligations to each other and by a common faith in the totem. Totemism is thus both a

contrary, it is certain that there have been profound changes in every direction among primitive races, so that it is never possible to decide without hesitation how far their present-day conditions and opinions preserve the primæval past in a petrified form and how far they are distortions and modifications of it. Hence arise the all-too-frequent disputes among the authorities as to which characteristics of a primitive civilization are to be regarded as primary and as to which are later and secondary developments. The determination of the original state of things thus invariably remains a matter of construction. Finally, it is not easy to feel one's way into primitive modes of thinking. We misunderstand primitive men just as easily as we do children, and we are always apt to interpret their actions and feelings according to our own mental constellations.

[1] *Totemism*, Edinburgh, 1887, reprinted in Frazer (1910, **1**, 3 ff.).

religious and a social system. In its religious aspect it consists of
the relations of mutual respect and protection between a man
and his totem; in its social aspect it consists of the relations of
the clansmen to each other and to men of other clans. In the
later history of totemism these two sides, the religious and the
social, tend to part company; the social system sometimes survives the religious; and, on the other hand, religion sometimes
bears traces of totemism in countries where the social system
based on totemism has disappeared. How in the origin of totemism these two sides were related to each other it is, in our ignorance of that origin, impossible to say with certainty. But on the
whole the evidence points strongly to the conclusion that the
two sides were originally inseparable; that, in other words, the
farther we go back, the more we should find that the clansman
regards himself and his totem as beings of the same species, and
the less he distinguishes between conduct towards his totem and
towards his fellow-clansmen.'

In giving particulars of totemism as a religious system, Frazer
begins by stating that the members of a totem clan call themselves by the name of their totem, and commonly believe themselves to be actually descended from it.[1] It follows from this
belief that they will not hunt the totem animal or kill or eat it
and, if it is something other than an animal, they refrain from
making use of it in other ways. The rules against killing or eating the totem are not the only taboos; sometimes they are forbidden to touch it, or even to look at it; in a number of cases the
totem may not be spoken of by its proper name. Any violation
of the taboos that protect the totem are automatically punished
by severe illness or death.[2]

Specimens of the totem animal are occasionally reared by
the clan and cared for in captivity.[3] A totem animal that is
found dead is mourned for and buried like a dead clansman. If
it is necessary to kill a totem animal, this is done according to a
prescribed ritual of apologies and ceremonies of expiation.

---

[1] [The last nine words are printed in spaced type in the original.]

[2] Cf. my earlier essay on taboo [above, p. 20].

[3] As is done to this day with the she-wolf in her cage beside the steps
leading up to the Capitol in Rome and with the bears in their den at
Berne.

The Return of Totemism in Childhood

The clan expects to receive protection and care from its totem. If it is a dangerous animal (such as a beast of prey or a venomous snake) there is a presumption that it will do no harm to its clansmen; and if that expectation is not fulfilled the injured man is expelled from the clan. Oaths, in Frazer's opinion, were originally ordeals; thus, many tests of descent and legitimacy were submitted for decision to the totem. The totem gives help in sickness and delivers omens and warnings to its clan. The appearance of the totem in or about a house is often regarded as an omen of death; the totem has come to fetch his kinsman.[1]

In particular important circumstances the clansman seeks to emphasize his kinship with the totem by making himself resemble it externally, by dressing in the skin of the animal, by incising a picture of the totem upon his own body, and so on. This identification with the totem is carried into effect in actions and words on the ceremonial occasions of birth, initiation and burial. Various magical and religious purposes are served by dances in which all the clansmen disguise themselves as their totem and imitate its behaviour. Lastly, there are ceremonies in which the totem animal is ceremoniously killed.[2]

The social aspect of totemism is principally expressed in a severely enforced injunction and a sweeping restriction.

The members of a totem clan are brothers and sisters and are bound to help and protect one another. If a member of a clan is killed by someone outside it, the whole clan of the aggressor is responsible for the deed and the whole clan of the murdered man is at one in demanding satisfaction for the blood that has been shed. The totem bond is stronger than that of the family in our sense. The two do not coincide, since the totem is as a rule inherited through the female line, and it is possible that paternal descent may originally have been left entirely out of account.

The corresponding taboo restriction prohibits members of the same totem clan from marrying or having sexual intercourse with each other. Here we have the notorious and mysterious correlate of totemism—exogamy. I have devoted the whole of the first essay in the present volume to that subject, so that here

[1] Like the White Lady in certain aristocratic families.
[2] Frazer (1910, **1**, 45). See my discussion of sacrifice below [p. 132 ff.].

I need only repeat that it originates from the intensification among savages of the horror of incest, that it would be fully explained as an assurance against incest under conditions of group marriage, and that it is primarily aimed at restraining the *younger* generation from incest and that only as a later development does it interfere with the older generation. [See above, pp. 4 and 9.]

To Frazer's account of totemism—one of the earliest in the literature of the subject—I will add a few extracts from one of the most recent ones. In his *Elemente der Völkerpsychologie*, Wundt (1912, 116 ff.) writes as follows: 'The totem animal is also usually regarded as the ancestral animal of the group in question. "Totem" is, on the one hand, a group name, and, on the other, a name indicative of ancestry. In the latter connection it has also a mythological significance. These various ideas, however, interplay in numerous ways. Some of the meanings may recede, so that totems have frequently become a mere nomenclature of tribal divisions, while at other times the idea of ancestry, or, perhaps also, the cult significance, predominates. . . .' The concept of the totem has a decisive influence upon tribal division and tribal organization, which are subject to certain norms of custom. 'These norms, and their fixed place in the beliefs and feelings of the tribal members, are connected with the fact that originally, at all events, the totem animal was regarded, for the most part, as having not merely given its name to a group of tribal members but as having actually been its forefather. . . . Bound up with this is the further fact that these animal ancestors possessed a cult. . . . Aside from specific ceremonies and ceremonial festivals, this animal cult originally found expression primarily in the relations maintained towards the totem animal. It was not merely a particular animal that was to a certain extent held sacred, but every representative of the species. The totem members were forbidden to eat the flesh of the totem animal, or were allowed to do so only under specific conditions. A significant counter-phenomenon, not irreconcilable with this, is the fact that on certain occasions the eating of the totem flesh constituted a sort of ceremony. . . .'

'. . . The most important social aspect of this totemic tribal organization, however, consists in the fact that it involved certain norms of custom regulating the intercourse of the separate groups with one another. Of these norms, those governing marriage relations were of first importance. The tribal organization of this period was bound up with an important institution, *exogamy*, which originated in the totemic age.' [English translation, 116 f.]

If we seek to penetrate to the original nature of totemism, without regard to subsequent accretions or attenuations, we find that its essential characteristics are these: Originally, all totems were animals, and were regarded as the ancestors of the different clans. Totems were inherited only through the female line. There was a prohibition against killing the totem (or—which, under primitive conditions, is the same thing—against eating it). Members of a totem clan were forbidden to practise sexual intercourse with one another.[1]

We shall now, perhaps, be struck by the fact that in Reinach's *Code du totémisme* one of the two principal taboos, that of exogamy, is not mentioned at all, while the belief upon which the second one is founded, namely descent from the totem animal, is only referred to in passing. My reason, however, for selecting the account given by Reinach (a writer, incidentally, who has made very valuable contributions to the subject) was to prepare

[1] [The last three sentences are printed in spaced type in the original.] The picture of totemism given by Frazer in his second work on the subject ('The Origin of Totemism', published in the *Fortnightly Review* in 1899) agrees with what I have written above: 'Thus, Totemism has commonly been treated as a primitive system both of religion and of society. As a system of religion it embraces the mystic union of the savage with his totem; as a system of society it comprises the relations in which men and women of the same totem stand to each other and to the members of other totemic groups. And corresponding to these two sides of the system are two rough and ready tests or canons of Totemism: first, the rule that a man may not kill or eat his totem animal or plant; and second, the rule that he may not marry or cohabit with a woman of the same totem.' [Reprinted in Frazer, 1910, 1, 101.] Frazer then proceeds (thus plunging us into the middle of the controversies on totemism): 'Whether the two sides—the religious and the social—have always co-existed or are essentially independent, is a question which has been variously answered.'

us for the differences of opinion between the authorities—differences into which we must now enter.

(2)

The more incontestible became the conclusion that totemism constitutes a regular phase in all cultures, the more urgent became the need for arriving at an understanding of it and for throwing light upon the puzzle of its essential nature. Everything connected with totemism seems to be puzzling: the decisive problems concern the origin of the idea of descent from the totem and the reasons for exogamy (or rather for the taboo upon incest of which exogamy is the expression), as well as the relation between these two institutions, totemic organization and prohibition of incest. Any satisfactory explanation should be at once an historical and a psychological one. It should tell us under what conditions this peculiar institution developed and to what psychical needs in men it has given expression.

My readers will, I am sure, be astonished to hear of the variety of angles from which attempts have been made to answer these questions, and of the wide divergences of opinion upon them put forward by the experts. Almost any generalization that could be made on the subject of totemism and exogamy seems open to question. Even the account that I have just given, derived from the book published by Frazer in 1887, is open to the criticism that it expresses the present writer's arbitrary preferences; and indeed it would be contested to-day by Frazer himself, who has repeatedly changed his opinions on the subject.[1]

It is plausible to suppose that an understanding of the essential nature of totemism and exogamy would best be arrived at, if it were possible to come nearer to the origins of the two institutions. But in this connection we must bear in mind Andrew

[1] He makes the following admirable comment upon such changes of opinion: 'That my conclusions on these difficult questions are final, I am not so foolish as to pretend. I have changed my views repeatedly, and I am resolved to change them again with every change of the evidence, for like a chameleon the candid inquirer should shift his colours with the shifting colours of the ground he treads.' (Frazer, 1910, **1**, xiii.)

The Return of Totemism in Childhood

Lang's warning that even primitive peoples have not retained the original forms of those institutions nor the conditions which gave rise to them; so that we have nothing whatever but hypotheses to fall back upon as a substitute for the observations which we are without.[1] Some of the attempted explanations seem, in the judgment of a psychologist, inadequate at the very outset: they are too rational and take no account of the emotional character of the matters to be explained. Others are based on assumptions which are unconfirmed by observation. Yet others rely upon material which would be better interpreted in another way. There is generally little difficulty in refuting the various views put forward: the authorities are as usual more effective in their criticisms of one another's work than in their own productions. The conclusion upon most of the points raised must be a *non liquet*. It is not surprising, therefore, that in the most recent literature on the subject (which is for the most part passed over in the present work) an unmistakable tendency emerges to reject any general solution of totemic problems as impracticable. (See, for instance, Goldenweiser, 1910.) In the discussion of these conflicting hypotheses which follows, I have ventured to disregard their chronological sequence.

(a) THE ORIGIN OF TOTEMISM

The question of the origin of totemism may be put in another way: how did it come about that primitive men called themselves (and their clans) after animals, plants and inanimate objects?[2]

McLennan (1865 and 1869–70), the Scot who discovered totemism and exogamy for the world of science, refrained from publishing any opinion on the origin of totemism. According to Andrew Lang (1905, 34) he was at one time inclined to think that it originated from the custom of tattooing. I propose to

---

[1] 'By the nature of the case, as the origin of totemism lies far beyond our powers of historical examination or of experiment, we must have recourse as regards this matter to conjecture.' (Lang, 1905, 27.) 'Nowhere do we see absolutely *primitive* man, and a totemic system in the making.' (Ibid., 29.)

[2] In the first instance probably after animals only.

divide the published theories on the origin of totemism into three groups—(α) the nominalist, (β) the sociological and (γ) the psychological.

(a) *Nominalist Theories*

My accounts of these theories will justify my having brought them together under the title I have adopted.

Garcilasso de la Vega, a descendant of the Peruvian Incas, who wrote a history of his people in the seventeenth century, seems already to have attributed the origin of what he knew of totemic phenomena to the need felt by clans to distinguish themselves from one another by the use of names. (Lang, 1905, 34.) Hundreds of years later the same idea was again proposed. Keane [1899, 396][1] regards totems as 'heraldic badges' by means of which individuals, families and clans sought to distinguish themselves from one another. The same idea is expressed once more by Max-Müller (1897 [1, 201]):[2] 'A totem is a clan mark, then a clan name, then the name of the ancestor of a clan, and lastly the name of something worshipped by a clan.' Julius Pikler,[3] writing later, declares: 'Mankind required both for communities and for individuals a permanent name which could be fixed in writing. . . . Thus totemism did not arise from the religious needs of men but from their practical, everyday needs. The core of totemism, nomenclature, is a result of the primitive technique of writing. In its nature a totem is like an easily drawn pictograph. But when once savages bore the name of an animal, they went on to form the idea of kinship with it.'

In the same way, Herbert Spencer (1870 and 1893, 331–346) regards the giving of names as the decisive factor in the origin of totemism. The personal characteristics of particular individuals, he argues, prompted the idea of calling them after animals, and in that way they acquired laudatory names or

[1] Quoted by Lang [1903, ix. f.].
[2] Quoted by Lang [1905, 118].
[3] Pikler and Somló [1900]. These authors justly describe their attempted explanation of the origin of totemism as 'a contribution to the materialist theory of history'.

nicknames which were handed on to their descendants. As a result of the vagueness and unintelligibility of primitive speech, later generations interpreted these names as evidence of descent from the actual animals. Totemism would thus be shown to be a misunderstood form of ancestor worship.

Lord Avebury (better known under his earlier name of Sir John Lubbock) gives a very similar account of the origin of totemism, though without insisting upon the element of misunderstanding. If, he says, we wish to explain animal-worship, we must not forget how often human names are borrowed from animals. The children and followers of a man who was called 'Bear' or 'Lion' naturally turned his name into a clan-name. Thence it came about that the animal itself would come to be regarded 'first with interest, then with respect and at length with a sort of awe'. [Lubbock, 1870, 171.]

What would seem to be an incontrovertible objection to this derivation of totem names from the names of individuals was brought forward by Fison.[1] He showed from conditions in Australia that the totem is invariably 'the badge of a group, not of an individual'. But even if this were not so, and the totem was originally the name of an individual, it could never—since totems are inherited through the female line—be transmitted to his children.

Moreover, the theories which I have so far discussed are obviously inadequate. They might perhaps explain the fact that primitive peoples adopt animal names for their clans, but they could never explain the importance that has become attached to this nomenclature—namely, the totemic system. The theory belonging to this group which most deserves attention is that proposed by Andrew Lang (1903 and 1905). He, too, regards the giving of names as the heart of the problem, but he introduces two interesting psychological factors and may thus claim to have led the way towards the final solution of the enigma of totemism.

Andrew Lang regards it as initially a matter of indifference how clans obtained their animal names. It is only necessary to assume that they awoke one day to the consciousness that they bore such names and could give no account of how this had

[1] Fison and Howitt (1880, 165), quoted by Lang (1905 [141]).

come about. The origin of the names had been forgotten.[1] They would then attempt to arrive at an explanation by speculating on the subject; and, in view of their belief in the importance of names, they were bound to reach all the ideas contained in the totemic system. Primitive races (as well as modern savages and even our own children[2]) do not, like us, regard names as something indifferent and conventional, but as significant and essential. A man's name is a principal component of his personality, perhaps even a portion of his soul. The fact of a primitive man bearing the same name as an animal must lead him to assume the existence of a mysterious and significant bond between himself and that particular species of animal. What other bond could it be than one of blood relationship? Once the similarity of names had led to this conclusion, the blood taboo would immediately involve all the totemic ordinances, including exogamy. 'No more than these three things—a group animal name of unknown origin; belief in a transcendental connection between all bearers, human and bestial, of the same name; and belief in the blood superstitions—was needed to give rise to all the totemic creeds and practices, including exogamy.' (Lang, 1905, 125 f.)

Lang's explanation falls into two parts. One part of it traces the totemic system as a matter of psychological necessity from the fact of the totems having animal names—always presupposing that the origin of these names had been forgotten. The second part of his theory goes on to try to explain how the names in fact originated; as we shall see, it is of a very different character from the first part.

This second part of Lang's theory differs in no essential way from the other theories which I have called 'nominalist'. The practical necessity for differentiation compelled the various clans to adopt names, and they therefore acquiesced in the names by which each clan was called by another clan. This 'naming from without' is the special feature of Lang's construction. The fact that the names adopted in this way were borrowed from animals needs no special comment and there is no reason why they should have been regarded in primitive times

[1] [This sentence is printed in spaced type by Freud.]
[2] See the discussion of taboo above, p. 54 ff.

as insulting or derisive. Moreover, Lang has adduced not a few instances from later historical times in which names that were originally given in derision by outsiders have been accepted and willingly adopted (e.g. '*Les Gueux*', 'Whigs' and 'Tories'). The hypothesis that in the course of time the origin of these names was forgotten connects this part of Lang's theory with the other part which I have already discussed.

(β) Sociological Theories

Reinach, who has been successful in tracing survivals of the totemic system in the cults and usages of later periods but who has always attached small importance to the factor of descent from the totem, remarks confidently in one passage that in his opinion totemism is nothing more than '*une hypertrophie de l'instinct social*'. (Reinach, 1905–12, **1**, 41.) A similar view seems to run through the recent book by Durkheim (1912). The totem, he argues, is the visible representative of social religion among the races concerned: it embodies the community, which is the true object of their worship.

Other writers have sought to find a more precise basis for the participation of the social instincts in the formation of totemic institutions. Thus Haddon (1902 [745])[1] supposes that each primitive clan originally subsisted upon some one species of animal or plant and perhaps traded in that particular article of food and exchanged it with other clans. It would inevitably follow that this clan would be known to the others by the name of the animal which was of such importance to it. At the same time the clan would be bound to become especially familiar with the animal and develop a peculiar interest in it, though this would be founded on no psychical motive other than the most elementary and urgent of human needs, that is, on hunger.

Against this most 'rational' of all the theories of totemism it has been objected that feeding conditions of this kind are never found among primitive races and have probably never existed. Savages are omnivorous, and the more so the lower their condition. Nor is it easy to see how an exclusive diet such as this could have developed into an almost religious attitude to the

[1] Quoted by Frazer (1910, **4**, 50).

totem, culminating in absolute abstention from the favourite food. [Cf. Frazer, 1910, **4**, 51.]

The first of the three theories on the origin of totemism which Frazer himself has supported at different times was a psychological one, and I shall deal with it later. His second theory, with which we are here concerned, took form under the influence of a momentous publication by two men who had made researches among the natives of Central Australia.

Spencer and Gillen (1899) described a number of peculiar observances, usages and beliefs found in a group of tribes known as the Arunta nation; and Frazer agreed with their opinion that these peculiarities were to be regarded as features of a primitive condition of things and might throw light upon the original and true meaning of totemism.

The peculiarities found in the Arunta tribe (a portion of the Arunta nation) are as follows:

(1) The Arunta are divided into totem clans, but the totem is not hereditary but determined for each individual in a manner to be described presently.

(2) The totem clans are not exogamous; but the restrictions upon marriage are based upon a highly developed division into marriage-classes, which have no connection with the totem.

(3) The function of the totem clans lies in their performing a ceremony which has as its aim the multiplication of the edible totem object by a characteristically magical method. (This ceremony is known as *intichiuma*.)

(4) The Arunta have a peculiar theory of conception and reincarnation. They believe that there are places scattered over the country ['totem centres'] at each of which the spirits of the dead of some one totem await reincarnation and enter the body of any woman who passes by the spot. When a child is born, the mother reports at which of these places she thinks it was conceived, and the child's totem is determined accordingly. It is further believed that the spirits (both of the dead and of the reborn) are intimately associated with certain peculiar stone amulets, known as *churinga*, which are found at these same centres.

Two factors seem to have led Frazer to suppose that the observances among the Arunta constitute the oldest form of totemism. First, there was the existence of certain myths which declared that the ancestors of the Arunta regularly ate their totem and always married women of their own totem. Secondly, there was the apparent disregard of the sexual act in their theory of conception. People who had not yet discovered that conception is the result of sexual intercourse might surely be regarded as the most backward and primitive of living men.

By focusing his judgment of totemism upon the *intichiuma* ceremony, Frazer came all at once to see the totemic system in an entirely new light: as a purely practical organization for meeting the most natural of human needs. (Cf. Haddon's theory above [p. 113].)[1] The system was simply an example upon a large scale of 'co-operative magic'. Primitive men set up what might be described as a magical producers' and consumers' union. Each totem clan undertook the business of guaranteeing the plentiful supply of one particular article of food. Where non-edible totems were concerned (such as dangerous animals, or rain, wind, etc.) the duty of the totem clan lay in controlling the natural force in question and in counteracting its injurious possibilities. The achievements of each clan were to the advantage of all the rest. Since each clan might eat none, or only very little, of its own totem, it provided that valuable material for the other clans and was itself provided in exchange with what *they* produced as their social totemic duty. In the light of the insight which he thus obtained from the *intichiuma* ceremony, Frazer came to believe that the prohibition against eating one's own totem had blinded people to the more important element in the situation, namely the injunction to produce as much as possible of an edible totem to meet the needs of other people.

Frazer accepted the Arunta tradition that each totem clan had originally eaten its own totem without restriction. But it was then difficult to understand the next stage in development, at which the clansmen became content with assuring a supply

[1] 'There is nothing vague or mystical about it, nothing of that metaphysical haze which some writers love to conjure up over the humble beginnings of human speculation, but which is utterly foreign to the simple, sensuous and concrete modes of thought of the savage.' (Frazer, 1910, **1**, 117.)

of the totem for others, while themselves renouncing its enjoyment almost completely. He supposed that this restriction had arisen, not from any kind of religious deference, but perhaps from observing that animals never fed upon their own kind: to do so might imply a breach in their identification with their totem and consequently reduce their power of controlling it. Or it might be that by sparing the creatures they hoped to conciliate them. Frazer, however, makes no disguise of the difficulties involved in these explanations (1910, **1**, 121 ff.): nor does he venture to suggest by what means the custom described in the Arunta myths of marrying within the totem was transformed into exogamy.

The theory based by Frazer on the *intichiuma* ceremony stands or falls with the assertion of the primitive character of the Arunta institutions. But in face of the objections raised by Durkheim[1] and Lang (1903 and 1905), that assertion appears untenable. On the contrary, the Arunta seem to be the most highly developed of the Australian tribes and to represent a stage of totemism in dissolution rather than its beginnings. The myths which impressed Frazer so deeply because, in contrast to the conditions that rule to-day, they lay stress upon liberty to eat the totem and to marry within the totem—these myths are easily explicable as wishful phantasies which, like the myth of a Golden Age, have been projected back into the past.

(γ) *Psychological Theories*

Frazer's first psychological theory, formed before he became acquainted with Spencer and Gillen's observations, was based on the belief in an 'external soul'.[2] The totem, according to this view, represented a safe place of refuge in which the soul could be deposited and so escape the dangers which threatened it. When a primitive man had deposited his soul in his totem he himself was invulnerable, and he naturally avoided doing any injury to the receptacle of his soul. Since, however, he did not

[1] In *L'année sociologique* (1898, 1902, 1905, etc.); see especially 'Sur le totémisme' (1902 [89 f.]).

[2] See Frazer: *The Golden Bough*, First Edition (1890), **2**, 332 ff. [Cf. also Frazer, 1910, **4**, 52 ff.]

know in which particular individual of the animal species concerned his own soul was lodged, it was reasonable for him to spare the whole species.

Frazer himself subsequently abandoned this theory that totemism was derived from a belief in souls; and, after coming to know of Spencer and Gillen's observations, adopted the sociological theory which I have already discussed. But he came to see himself that the motive from which that second theory derived totemism was too 'rational' and that it implied a social organization which was too complicated to be described as primitive.[1] The magical co-operative societies now seemed to him to be the fruit rather than the seed of totemism. He sought for some simpler factor, some primitive superstition behind these structures, to which the origin of totemism might be traced back. At last he found this original factor in the Arunta's remarkable story of conception.

The Arunta, as I have already explained, eliminate the connection between the sexual act and conception. At the moment at which a woman feels she is a mother, a spirit, which has been awaiting reincarnation in the nearest totem centre where the spirits of the dead collect, has entered her body. She will bear this spirit as a child, and the child will have the same totem as all the spirits waiting at that particular centre. This theory of conception cannot explain totemism, since it presupposes the existence of totems. But let us go back a step further and suppose that originally the woman believed that the animal, plant, stone or other object, with which her imagination was occupied at the moment when she first felt she was a mother, actually made its way into her and was later born in human form. In that case the identity between a man and his totem would have a factual basis in his mother's belief and all the remaining totem ordinances (with the exception of exogamy) would follow. A man would refuse to eat this animal or plant because to do so would amount to eating himself. He would, however, have a reason for occasionally partaking of his totem in a ceremonial

---

[1] 'It is unlikely that a community of savages should deliberately parcel out the realm of nature into provinces, assign each province to a particular band of magicians, and bid all the bands to work their magic and weave their spells for the common good.' (Frazer, 1910, 4, 57.)

manner, because in that way he might strengthen his identification with the totem, which is the essence of totemism. Some observations made by Rivers [1909, 173 f.] upon the natives of the Banks' Islands¹ seemed to prove a direct identification of human beings with their totem on the basis of a similar theory of conception.

Accordingly, the ultimate source of totemism would be the savages' ignorance of the process by which men and animals reproduce their kind; and, in particular, ignorance of the part played by the male in fertilization. This ignorance must have been facilitated by the long interval between the act of fertilization and the birth of the child (or the first perception of its movements). Thus totemism would be a creation of the feminine rather than of the masculine mind: its roots would lie in 'the sick fancies of pregnant women'. 'Anything indeed that struck a woman at that mysterious moment of her life when she first knows herself to be a mother might easily be identified by her with the child in her womb. Such maternal fancies, so natural and seemingly so universal, appear to be the root of totemism.' (Frazer, 1910, **4**, 63.)

The main objection to this third of Frazer's theories is the same as has already been brought against the second or sociological one. The Arunta seem to be far removed from the beginnings of totemism. Their denial of paternity does not appear to rest upon primitive ignorance; in some respects they themselves make use of descent through the father. They seem to have sacrificed paternity for the sake of some sort of speculation designed to honour the souls of their ancestors.² They have enlarged the myth of the impregnation of a virgin by the spirit into a general theory of conception; but that is no reason why ignorance of the conditions governing fertilization should be imputed to them any more than to the peoples of antiquity at the time of the origin of the Christian myths.

Another psychological theory of the origin of totemism has been advanced by a Dutchman, G. A. Wilken [1884, 997]. It connects totemism with the belief in the transmigration of souls. 'The animal in which the souls of the dead are thought by pre-

¹ Quoted by Frazer (1910, **2**, 89 ff. and **4**, 59).
² 'That belief is a philosophy far from primitive.' (Lang, 1905, 192.)

ference to be incarnate becomes a kinsman, an ancestor, and as such is revered.'[1] It seems more likely, however, that the belief in transmigration was derived from totemism than vice versa.

Yet another theory of totemism is held by some eminent American ethnologists, Franz Boas, C. Hill-Tout, and others. It is based upon observations on North American Indian totemic clans and maintains that the totem was originally the guardian spirit of an ancestor, who acquired it in a dream and transmitted it to his descendants. We have already heard the difficulties which stand in the way of the view that totems are inherited from single individuals [cf. p. 111]; but apart from this, the Australian evidence lends no support to the theory that totems are derived from guardian spirits. (Frazer, 1910, 4, 48 ff.)

The last of the psychological theories, that put forward by Wundt (1912, 190), is based upon two facts. 'In the first place, the original totem, and the one which continues to remain most common, is the animal; and, secondly, the earliest totem animals are identical with soul animals.' [English translation, 192.] Soul animals (such as birds, snakes, lizards and mice) are appropriate receptacles of souls which have left the body, on account of their rapid movements or flight through the air or of other qualities likely to produce surprise or alarm. Totem animals are derived from the transformations of the 'breath-soul' into animals. Thus, according to Wundt, totemism is directly connected with the belief in spirits, that is to say with animism.

(*b*) and (*c*) THE ORIGIN OF EXOGAMY AND ITS RELATION TO TOTEMISM

I have set out the different theories about totemism in some detail. But even so, compression has been inevitable and I fear that my account may have suffered in consequence. In what follows, however, I shall venture, for my readers' sake, to be still more condensed. The discussions on the exogamy practised by totemic peoples are, owing to the nature of the material with which they deal, particularly complicated and diffuse—one might even say confused. The purposes of the present work make it possible for me to limit myself to tracing certain of the

[1] Quoted by Frazer (1910, 4, 45 f.).

main lines of dispute, while referring those who wish to enter into the subject more deeply to the specialized writings from which I have so frequently quoted.

The attitude taken by an author on the problems of exogamy must naturally depend to some extent on the position he has adopted towards the various theories of totemism. Some of the explanations of totemism exclude any connection with exogamy, so that the two institutions fall completely apart. Thus we find two opposing views: one which seeks to maintain the original presumption that exogamy forms an inherent part of the totemic system, and the other which denies that there is any such connection and holds that the convergence between these two features of the oldest cultures is a chance one. This latter opinion has been adopted without qualification by Frazer in his later works: 'I must request the reader to bear constantly in mind', he writes, 'that the two institutions of totemism and exogamy are fundamentally distinct in origin and nature, though they have accidentally crossed and blended in many tribes.' (Frazer, 1910, **1**, xii.) He gives an explicit warning that the opposite view must be a source of endless difficulties and misunderstandings.

Other writers have, on the contrary, found a means of regarding exogamy as an inevitable consequence of the basic principles of totemism. Durkheim (1898, 1902 and 1905) has put forward the view that the taboo attached to totems was bound to involve prohibition against practising sexual intercourse with a woman of the same totem. The totem is of the same blood as the man and consequently the ban upon shedding blood (in connection with defloration and menstruation) prohibits him from sexual relations with a woman belonging to his totem.[1] Andrew Lang (1905, 125), who agrees with Durkheim on this subject, believes that the prohibition against women of the same clan might operate even without any blood taboo. The general totem taboo (which, for instance, forbids a man to sit under his own totem tree) would, in Lang's opinion, have been sufficient. Incidentally, he complicates this with another explanation of exogamy (see below [p. 126]) and omits to show how the two explanations are related to each other.

[1] See the criticisms of Durkheim's views by Frazer (1910, **4**, 100 ff.).

The Return of Totemism in Childhood

As regards the chronological relations between the two institutions, most of the authorities agree that totemism is the older of them and that exogamy arose later.[1]

Of the theories which seek to show that exogamy is independent of totemism I shall only draw attention to a few which throw light on the attitude of the different authors to the problem of incest.

McLennan (1865) ingeniously inferred the existence of exogamy from the vestiges of customs which seemed to indicate the earlier practice of marriage by capture. He formed a hypothesis that in the earliest times it had been a general usage for men to obtain their wives from another group and that marriage with a woman of their own group gradually 'came to be considered improper because it was unusual' [ibid., 289]. He accounted for the prevalence of exogamy by supposing that the practice of killing the majority of female children at birth had led to a scarcity of women in primitive societies. We are not here concerned with the question of how far these assumptions of McLennan's are supported by the actual findings. What interests us far more is the fact that his hypotheses fail to explain why the male members of a group should refuse themselves access to the few remaining women of their own blood—the fact that he entirely overlooks the problem of incest. (Frazer, 1910, **4**, 71–92.)

Other students of exogamy, on the contrary, and evidently with greater justice, have seen in exogamy an institution for the prevention of incest.[2] When one considers the gradually increasing complication of the Australian restrictions upon marriage, it is impossible not to accept the opinions of Morgan (1877), Frazer (1910, **4**, 105 ff.), Howitt [1904, 143] and Baldwin Spencer that those regulations bear (in Frazer's words) 'the impress of deliberate design' and that they aimed at achieving the result they have in fact achieved. 'In no other way does it seem possible to explain in all its details a system at once so complex and so regular.' (Frazer, ibid., 106.)

It is interesting to observe that the first restrictions produced

[1] See, for instance, Frazer (1910, **4**, 75): 'The totemic clan is a totally different social organism from the exogamous clan, and we have good grounds for thinking that it is far older.'

[2] Cf. the first essay in this book.

by the introduction of marriage classes affected the sexual freedom of the *younger* generation (that is, incest between brothers and sisters and between sons and mothers) whereas incest between fathers and daughters was only prevented by a further extension of the regulations.

But the fact that exogamous sexual restrictions were imposed intentionally throws no light on the motive which led to their imposition. What is the ultimate source of the horror of incest which must be recognized as the root of exogamy? To explain it by the existence of an instinctive dislike of sexual intercourse with blood relatives—that is to say, by an appeal to the fact that there *is* a horror of incest—is clearly unsatisfactory; for social experience shows that, in spite of this supposed instinct, incest is no uncommon event even in our present-day society, and history tells us of cases in which incestuous marriage between privileged persons was actually the rule.

Westermarck (1906–8, **2**, 368)[1] has explained the horror of incest on the ground that 'there is an innate aversion to sexual intercourse between persons living very closely together from early youth, and that, as such persons are in most cases related by blood, this feeling would naturally display itself in custom and law as a horror of intercourse between near kin'. Havelock Ellis [1914, 205 f.], though he disputed the instinctiveness of the aversion, subscribed to this explanation in the main: 'The normal failure of the pairing instinct to manifest itself in the case of brothers and sisters, or of boys and girls brought up together from infancy, is a merely negative phenomenon due to the inevitable absence in those circumstances of the conditions which evoke the pairing instinct. . . . Between those who have been brought up together from childhood all the sensory stimuli of vision, hearing and touch have been dulled by use, trained to the calm level of affection, and deprived of their potency to arouse the erethistic excitement which produces sexual tumescence.'

It seems to me very remarkable that Westermarck should consider that this innate aversion to sexual intercourse with those with whom one has been intimate in childhood is also the

[1] In the same chapter he replies to various objections which have been raised against his views.

equivalent in psychical terms of the biological fact that in-breeding is detrimental to the species. A biological instinct of the kind suggested would scarcely have gone so far astray in its psychological expression that, instead of applying to blood-relatives (intercourse with whom might be injurious to repro-duction), it affected persons who were totally innocuous in this respect, merely because they shared a common home. I cannot resist referring, too, to Frazer's admirable criticism of Wester-marck's theory. Frazer finds it inexplicable that to-day there should be scarcely any sexual aversion to intercourse with house-mates, whereas the horror of incest, which on Wester-marck's theory is only a derivative of that aversion, should have increased so enormously. But some further comments of Frazer's go deeper, and these I shall reproduce in full, since they are in essential agreement with the arguments which I put forward in my essay on taboo:

'It is not easy to see why any deep human instinct should need to be reinforced by law. There is no law commanding men to eat and drink or forbidding them to put their hands in the fire. Men eat and drink and keep their hands out of the fire in-stinctively for fear of natural not legal penalties, which would be entailed by violence done to these instincts. The law only forbids men to do what their instincts incline them to do; what nature itself prohibits and punishes, it would be superfluous for the law to prohibit and punish. Accordingly we may always safely assume that crimes forbidden by law are crimes which many men have a natural propensity to commit. If there was no such propensity there would be no such crimes, and if no such crimes were committed what need to forbid them? Instead of assuming, therefore, from the legal prohibition of incest that there is a natural aversion to incest, we ought rather to assume that there is a natural instinct in favour of it, and that if the law represses it, as it represses other natural instincts, it does so be-cause civilized men have come to the conclusion that the satis-faction of these natural instincts is detrimental to the general interests of society.' (Frazer, 1910, **4**, 97 f.)

I may add to these excellent arguments of Frazer's that the findings of psycho-analysis make the hypothesis of an innate aversion to incestuous intercourse totally untenable. They have shown, on the contrary, that the earliest sexual excitations of youthful human beings are invariably of an incestuous character and that such impulses when repressed play a part that can scarcely be over-estimated as motive forces of neuroses in later life.

Thus the view which explains the horror of incest as an innate instinct must be abandoned. Nor can anything more favourable be said of another, widely held explanation of the law against incest, according to which primitive peoples noticed at an early date the dangers with which their race was threatened by inbreeding and for that reason deliberately adopted the prohibition. There are a host of objections to this theory. (Cf. Durkheim, 1898 [33 ff.].) Not only must the prohibition against incest be older than any domestication of animals which might have enabled men to observe the effects of inbreeding upon racial characters, but even to-day the detrimental results of inbreeding are not established with certainty and cannot easily be demonstrated in man. Moreover, everything that we know of contemporary savages makes it highly improbable that their most remote ancestors were already concerned with the question of preserving their later progeny from injury. Indeed it is almost absurd to attribute to such improvident creatures motives of hygiene and eugenics to which consideration is scarcely paid in our own present-day civilization.[1]

Lastly, account must be taken of the fact that a prohibition against inbreeding, based upon practical motives of hygiene, on the ground of its tending to racial enfeeblement, seems quite inadequate to explain the profound abhorrence shown towards incest in our society. As I have shown elsewhere,[2] this feeling seems to be even more active and intense among contemporary primitive peoples than among civilized ones.

It might have been expected that here again we should have before us a choice between sociological, biological and psychological explanations. (In this connection the psychological motives should perhaps be regarded as representing biological forces.) Nevertheless, at the end of our inquiry, we can only sub-

[1] Darwin [1875, 2, 127] writes of savages that they 'are not likely to reflect on distant evils to their progeny'.
[2] See the first essay in this volume [p. 9].

scribe to Frazer's resigned conclusion. We are ignorant of the origin of the horror of incest and cannot even tell in what direction to look for it. None of the solutions of the enigma that have been proposed seems satisfactory.[1]

I must, however, mention one other attempt at solving it. It is of a kind quite different from any that we have so far considered, and might be described as 'historical'.

This attempt is based upon an hypothesis of Charles Darwin's upon the social state of primitive men. Darwin deduced from the habits of the higher apes that men, too, originally lived in comparatively small groups or hordes[2] within which the jealousy of the oldest and strongest male prevented sexual promiscuity. 'We may indeed conclude from what we know of the jealousy of all male quadrupeds, armed, as many of them are, with special weapons for battling with their rivals, that promiscuous intercourse in a state of nature is extremely improbable. . . . Therefore, if we look far enough back in the stream of time, . . . judging from the social habits of man as he now exists . . . the most probable view is that primæval man aboriginally lived in small communities, each with as many wives as he could support and obtain, whom he would have jealously guarded against all other men. Or he may have lived with several wives by himself, like the Gorilla; for all the natives "agree that but one adult male is seen in a band; when the young male grows up, a contest takes place for mastery, and the strongest, by killing and driving out the others, establishes himself as the head of the community." (Dr. Savage, in *Boston Journal of Nat. Hist.*, vol. v, 1845-7, p. 423.) The younger males, being thus expelled and wandering about, would, when at last successful in finding a partner, prevent too close interbreeding within the limits of the same family.' (Darwin, 1871, **2**, 362 f.)

[1] 'Thus the ultimate origin of exogamy, and with it of the law of incest—since exogamy was devised to prevent incest—remains a problem nearly as dark as ever.' (Frazer, 1910, **1**, 165.)

[2] [Freud's use, here and subsequently, of the word 'horde' may give rise to confusion. In ordinary English usage 'horde' suggests a very large and unorganized mass of people. The present context makes it plain that Freud uses the word to denote a more or less organized group of limited size—what Atkinson terms 'the cyclopean family'.]

Atkinson (1903) seems to have been the first to realize that the practical consequence of the conditions obtaining in Darwin's primal horde must be exogamy for the young males. Each of them might, after being driven out, establish a similar horde, in which the same prohibition upon sexual intercourse would rule owing to its leader's jealousy. In course of time this would produce what grew into a conscious law: 'No sexual relations between those who share a common home.' After the establishment of totemism this regulation would assume another form and would run: 'No sexual relations within the totem.'

Andrew Lang (1905, 114 and 143) accepted this explanation of exogamy. In the same volume, however, he supports the other theory (held by Durkheim), according to which exogamy was a resultant of the totemic laws. [Cf. p. 120.] It is a little difficult to bring these two points of view into harmony: according to the first theory exogamy would have originated before totemism, while according to the second it would have been derived from it.[1]

(3)

Into this obscurity one single ray of light is thrown by psycho-analytic observation.

There is a great deal of resemblance between the relations of children and of primitive men towards animals. Children show no trace of the arrogance which urges adult civilized men to

[1] 'If it be granted that exogamy existed in practice, on the lines of Mr. Darwin's theory, before the totem beliefs lent to the practice a *sacred* sanction, our task is relatively easy. The first practical rule would be that of the jealous Sire, "No males to touch the females in my camp", with expulsion of adolescent sons. *In efflux of time that rule, become habitual,* would be, "No marriage within the local group". Next, let the local groups receive names, such as Emus, Crows, Opossums, Snipes, and the rule becomes, "No marriage within the local group of animal name; no Snipe to marry Snipe." But, if the primal groups were not exogamous, they would become so, as soon as totemic myths and tabus were developed out of the animal, vegetable, and other names of local groups.' (Lang, 1905, 143.) (The italics in the middle of this passage are mine.) In his last discussion of this subject, moreover, Lang (1911 [404]) states that he has 'abandoned the idea that exogamy is a consequence of the general totemic taboo'.

draw a hard-and-fast line between their own nature and that of all other animals. Children have no scruples over allowing animals to rank as their full equals. Uninhibited as they are in the avowal of their bodily needs, they no doubt feel themselves more akin to animals than to their elders, who may well be a puzzle to them.

Not infrequently, however, a strange rift occurs in the excellent relations between children and animals. A child will suddenly begin to be frightened of some particular species of animal and to avoid touching or seeing any individual of that species. The clinical picture of an animal phobia emerges—a very common, and perhaps the earliest, form of psycho-neurotic illness occurring in childhood. As a rule the phobia is attached to animals in which the child has hitherto shown a specially lively interest and it has nothing to do with any particular individual animal. There is no large choice of animals that may become objects of a phobia in the case of children living in towns: horses, dogs, cats, less often birds, and with striking frequency very small creatures such as beetles and butterflies. The senseless and immoderate fear shown in these phobias is sometimes attached to animals only known to the child from picture books and fairy tales. On a few rare occasions it is possible to discover what has led to an unusual choice of this kind; and I have to thank Karl Abraham for telling me of a case in which the child himself explained that his fear of wasps was due to their colour and stripes reminding him of tigers, which from all accounts were beasts to be feared.[1]

No detailed analytic examination has yet been made of children's animal phobias, though they would greatly repay study. This neglect has no doubt been due to the difficulty of analysing children of such a tender age. It cannot therefore be claimed that we know the general meaning of these disorders and I myself am of the opinion that this may not turn out to be of a uniform nature. But a few cases of phobias of this kind directed towards the larger animals have proved accessible to analysis and have thus yielded their secret to the investigator. It was the same in every case: where the children concerned were boys,

[1] [Subsequently published. (Abraham, 1914, 82; English translation, 228.)]

their fear related at bottom to their father and had merely been displaced on to the animal.

Everyone with psycho-analytic experience will no doubt have come across cases of the sort and have derived the same impression from them. Yet I can quote only a few detailed publications on the subject. This paucity of literature is an accidental circumstance and it must not be supposed that our conclusions are based on a few scattered observations. I may mention, for instance, a writer who has studied the neuroses of childhood with great understanding—Dr. M. Wulff, of Odessa.[1] In the course of a case-history of a nine-year-old boy he reports that at the age of four the patient had suffered from a dog-phobia. 'When he saw a dog running past in the street, he would weep and call out: "Dear doggie, don't bite me! I'll be good!" By "being good" he meant "not playing on the fiddle" '—not masturbating. (Wulff, 1912, 15.) 'The boy's dog-phobia', the author explains, 'was in reality his fear of his father displaced on to dogs; for his curious exclamation "Doggie, I'll be good!"— that is, "I won't masturbate"—was directed to his father, who had forbidden him to masturbate.' Wulff adds a footnote which is in complete agreement with my views and at the same time bears witness to the frequent occurrence of such experiences: 'Phobias of this type (phobias of horses, dogs, cats, fowls and other domestic animals) are, in my opinion, at least as common in childhood as *pavor nocturnus*; and in analysis they almost invariably turn out to be a displacement on to the animals of the child's fear of one of his parents. I should not be prepared to maintain that the same mechanism applies to the widespread phobias of rats and mice.' [Ibid., 16.]

I recently published (1909a) an 'Analysis of a Phobia in a Five-Year-Old Boy', the material of which was supplied to me by the little patient's father. The boy had a phobia of horses, and as a result he refused to go out in the street. He expressed a fear that the horse would come into the room and bite him; and it turned out that this must be the punishment for a wish that the horse might fall down (that is, die). After the boy's fear of his father had been removed by reassurances, it became evident that he was struggling against wishes which had as their subject

[1] [Later Dr. M. Woolf of Tel-Aviv.]

the idea of his father being absent (going away on a journey, dying). He regarded his father (as he made all too clear) as a competitor for the favours of his mother, towards whom the obscure foreshadowings of his budding sexual wishes were aimed. Thus he was situated in the typical attitude of a male child towards his parents to which we have given the name of the 'Œdipus complex' and which we regard in general as the nuclear complex of the neuroses. The new fact that we have learnt from the analysis of 'little Hans'—a fact with an important bearing upon totemism—is that in such circumstances children displace some of their feelings from their father on to an animal.

Analysis is able to trace the associative paths along which this displacement passes—both the fortuitous paths and those with a significant content. Analysis also enables us to discover the *motives* for the displacement. The hatred of his father that arises in a boy from rivalry for his mother is not able to achieve uninhibited sway over his mind; it has to contend against his old-established affection and admiration for the very same person. The child finds relief from the conflict arising out of this double-sided, this ambivalent emotional attitude towards his father by displacing his hostile and fearful feelings on to a *substitute* for his father. The displacement cannot, however, bring the conflict to an end, it cannot effect a clear-cut severance between the affectionate and the hostile feelings. On the contrary, the conflict is resumed in relation to the object on to which the displacement has been made: the ambivalence is extended to *it*. There could be no doubt that little Hans was not only *frightened* of horses; he also approached them with admiration and interest. As soon as his anxiety began to diminish, he identified himself with the dreaded creature: he began to jump about like a horse and in his turn bit his father.[1] At another stage in the resolution of his phobia he did not hesitate to identify his parents with some other large animals.[2]

It may fairly be said that in these children's phobias some of the features of totemism reappear, but reversed into their negative. We are, however, indebted to Ferenczi (1913*a*) for an in-

[1] Freud (1909*a* [English translation, 194]).
[2] In his giraffe phantasy [ibid., 179–82].

teresting history of a single case which can only be described as an instance of *positive* totemism in a child. It is true that in the case of little Árpád (the subject of Ferenczi's report) his totemic interests did not arise in direct relation with his Œdipus complex but on the basis of its narcissistic precondition, the fear of castration. But any attentive reader of the story of little Hans will find abundant evidence that he, too, admired his father as possessing a big penis and feared him as threatening his own. The same part is played by the father alike in the Œdipus and the castration complexes—the part of a dreaded enemy to the sexual interests of childhood. The punishment which he threatens is castration, or its substitute, blinding.[1]

When little Árpád was two and a half years old, he had once, while he was on a summer holiday, tried to micturate into the fowl-house and a fowl had bitten or snapped at his penis. A year later, when he was back in the same place, he himself turned into a fowl; his one interest was in the fowl-house and in what went on there and he abandoned human speech in favour of cackling and crowing. At the time at which the observation was made (when he was five years old) he had recovered his speech, but his interests and his talk were entirely concerned with chickens and other kinds of poultry. They were his only toys and he only sang songs that had some mention of fowls in them. His attitude towards his totem animal was superlatively ambivalent: he showed both hatred and love to an extravagant degree. His favourite game was playing slaughtering fowls. 'The slaughtering of poultry was a regular festival for him. He would dance round the animals' bodies for hours at a time in a state of intense excitement.'[1] But afterwards he would kiss and stroke the slaughtered animal or would clean and caress the toy fowls that he had himself ill-treated.

Little Árpád himself saw to it that the meaning of his strange behaviour should not remain hidden. From time to time he translated his wishes from the totemic language into that of everyday life. 'My father's the cock', he said on one occasion,

---

[1] For the substitution of blinding for castration—a substitution that occurs, too, in the myth of Œdipus—see Reitler (1913), Ferenczi (1913*b*), Rank (1913) and Eder (1913).

[1] [Ferenczi, 1913*a* (English translation, 246.)]

and another time: 'Now I'm small, now I'm a chicken. When I get bigger I'll be a fowl. When I'm bigger still I'll be a cock.' On another occasion he suddenly said he would like to eat some 'fricassee of mother' (on the analogy of fricassee of chicken). [Ibid., 249.] He was very generous in threatening other people with castration, just as he himself had been threatened with it for his masturbatory activities.

There was no doubt, according to Ferenczi, as to the sources of Árpád's interest in events in the poultry-yard: 'the continual sexual activity between the cock and hens, the laying of eggs and the hatching out of the young brood' gratified his sexual curiosity, the real object of which was *human* family-life. [Ibid., 250.] He showed that he had formed his own choice of sexual objects on the model of life in the hen-run, for he said one day to the neighbour's wife: 'I'll marry you and your sister and my three cousins and the cook; no, not the cook, I'll marry my mother instead.' [Ibid., 252.]

Later on we shall be able to assess the worth of this observation more completely. At the moment I will only emphasize two features in it which offer valuable points of agreement with totemism: the boy's complete identification with his totem animal[1] and his ambivalent emotional attitude to it. These observations justify us, in my opinion, in substituting the father for the totem animal in the formula for totemism (in the case of males). It will be observed that there is nothing new or particularly daring in this step forward. Indeed, primitive men say the very same thing themselves, and, where the totemic system is still in force to-day, they describe the totem as their common ancestor and primal father. All we have done is to take at its literal value an expression used by these people, of which the anthropologists have been able to make very little and which they have therefore been glad to keep in the background. Psycho-analysis, on the contrary, leads us to put special stress upon this same point and to take it as the starting-point of our attempt at explaining totemism.[2]

---

[1] This, according to Frazer (1910, 4, 5), constitutes 'the whole essence of totemism': 'totemism is an identification of a man with his totem.'

[2] I have to thank Otto Rank for bringing to my notice a dog-phobia in an intelligent young man. His explanation of the way in which he

Totem and Taboo

The first consequence of our substitution is most remarkable. If the totem animal is the father, then the two principal ordinances of totemism, the two taboo prohibitions which constitute its core—not to kill the totem and not to have sexual relations with a woman of the same totem—coincide in their content with the two crimes of Œdipus, who killed his father and married his mother, as well as with the two primal wishes of children, the insufficient repression or the re-awakening of which forms the nucleus of perhaps every psychoneurosis. If this equation is anything more than a misleading trick of chance, it must enable us to throw a light upon the origin of totemism in the inconceivably remote past. In other words, it would enable us to make it probable that the totemic system—like little Hans's animal phobia and little Arpád's poultry perversion—was a product of the conditions involved in the Œdipus complex. In order to pursue this possibility, we shall have, in the following pages, to study a feature of the totemic system (or, as we might say, of the totemic religion) which I have hitherto scarcely found an opportunity of mentioning.

(4)

William Robertson Smith, who died in 1894—physicist, philologist, Bible critic and archæologist—was a man of many-sided interests, clear-sighted and liberal-minded. In his book on the *Religion of the Semites* (first published in 1889)[1] he put forward the hypothesis that a peculiar ceremony known as the 'totem meal' had from the very first formed an integral part of the totemic system. At that time he had only a single piece of evidence in support of his theory: an account of a procedure of the kind dating from the fifth century A.D. But by an analysis of the nature of sacrifice among the ancient Semites he was able to lend his hypothesis a high degree of probability. Since sacrifice implies a divinity, it was a question of arguing back from a com-

acquired his illness sounds markedly like the totemic theory of the Arunta which I mentioned on page 114: he thought he had heard from his father that his mother had had a severe fright from a dog during her pregnancy.

[1] [The second and revised edition, which is the one here quoted, appeared posthumously in 1894.]

132

paratively high phase of religious ritual to the lowest one, that is, to totemism.

I will now attempt to extract from Robertson Smith's admirable work those of his statements on the origin and meaning of the ritual of sacrifice which are of decisive interest for us. In so doing I must omit all the details, often so fascinating, and neglect all the later developments. It is quite impossible for an epitome such as this to give my readers any notion of the lucidity and convincing force of the original.

Robertson Smith [1894, 214] explains that sacrifice at the altar was the essential feature in the ritual of ancient religions. It plays the same part in all religions, so that its origin must be traced back to very general causes, operating everywhere in the same manner. Sacrifice—the sacred act *par excellence* (*sacrificium, ἱερουργία*)—originally had a somewhat different meaning, however, from its later one of making an offering to the deity in order to propitiate him or gain his favour. (The non-religious usage of the word followed from this subsidiary sense of 'renunciation'. [See below, p. 150.]) It can be shown that, to begin with, sacrifice was nothing other than 'an act of fellowship between the deity and his worshippers'. [Ibid., 224.]

The materials offered for sacrifice were things that can be eaten or drunk; men sacrificed to their deity the things on which they themselves lived: flesh, cereals, fruit, wine and oil. Only in the case of flesh were there limitations and exceptions. The god shared the animal sacrifices with his worshippers, the vegetable offerings were for him alone. There is no doubt that animal sacrifices were the older and were originally the only ones. Vegetable sacrifices arose from the offering of first-fruits and were in the nature of a tribute to the lord of the earth and of the land; but animal sacrifices are more ancient than agriculture. [Ibid., 222.]

Linguistic survivals make it certain that the portion of the sacrifice allotted to the god was originally regarded as being literally his food. As the nature of gods grew progressively less material, this conception became a stumbling-block. It was avoided by assigning to the deity only the *liquid* part of the meal. Later, the use of fire, which caused the flesh of the sacrifice upon the altar to rise in smoke, afforded a method of dealing with human food more appropriate to the divine mature. [Ibid., 224, 229.] The drink-offering consisted originally of the blood of the animal victim. This was later replaced by wine. In ancient times wine was regarded as 'the blood of the grape', and it has been so described by modern poets. [Ibid., 230.]

The oldest form of sacrifice, then, older than the use of fire or the knowledge of agriculture, was the sacrifice of animals, whose flesh and blood were enjoyed in common by the god and his worshippers. It was essential that each one of the participants should have his share of the meal.

A sacrifice of this kind was a public ceremony, a festival celebrated by the whole clan. Religion in general was an affair of the community and religious duty was a part of social obligation. Everywhere a sacrifice involves a feast and a feast cannot be celebrated without a sacrifice. The sacrificial feast was an occasion on which individuals rose joyously above their own interests and stressed the mutual dependence existing between one another and their god. [Ibid., 255.]

The ethical force of the public sacrificial meal rested upon very ancient ideas of the significance of eating and drinking together. Eating and drinking with a man was a symbol and a confirmation of fellowship and mutual social obligations. What was *directly* expressed by the sacrificial meal was only the fact that the god and his worshippers were 'commensals',[1] but every other point in their mutual relations was included in this. Customs still in force among the Arabs of the desert show that what is binding in a common meal is not a religious factor but the act of eating itself. Anyone who has eaten the smallest morsel of food with one of these Bedouin or has swallowed a mouthful of his milk need no longer fear him as an enemy but may feel secure in his protection and help. Not, however, for an unlimited time; strictly speaking, only so long as the food which has been eaten in common remains in the body. Such was the realistic view of the bond of union. It needed repetition in order to be confirmed and made permanent. [Ibid., 269–70.]

But why is this binding force attributed to eating and drinking together? In primitive societies there was only one kind of bond which was absolute and inviolable—that of kinship. The

[1] [I.e. that they sat at one table.]

solidarity of such a fellowship was complete. 'A kin was a group of persons whose lives were so bound up together, in what must be called a physical unity, that they could be treated as parts of one common life. . . . In a case of homicide Arabian tribesmen do not say, "The blood of M. or N. has been spilt", naming the man; they say, "Our blood has been spilt". In Hebrew the phrase by which one claims kinship is "I am your bone and your flesh". ' Thus kinship implies participation in a common substance. It is therefore natural that it is not merely based on the fact that a man is a part of his mother's substance, having been born of her and having been nourished by her milk, but that it can be acquired and strengthened by food which a man eats later and with which his body is renewed. If a man shared a meal with his god he was expressing a conviction that they were of one substance; and he would never share a meal with one whom he regarded as a stranger. [Ibid., 273–5.]

The sacrificial meal, then, was originally a feast of kinsmen, in accordance with the law that only kinsmen eat together. In our own society the members of a family have their meals in common; but the sacrificial meal bears no relation to the family. Kinship is an older thing than family life, and in the most primitive societies known to us the family contained members of more than one kindred. The man married a woman of another clan and the children inherited their mother's clan; so that there was no communion of kin between the man and the other members of the family. In a family of such a kind there was no common meal. To this day, savages eat apart and alone and the religious food prohibitions of totemism often make it impossible for them to eat in common with their wives and children. [Ibid., 277–8.]

Let us now turn to the sacrificial animal. As we have heard, there is no gathering of a clan without an animal sacrifice, nor —and this now becomes significant—any slaughter of an animal except upon these ceremonial occasions. While game and the milk of domestic animals might be consumed without any qualms, religious scruples made it impossible to kill a domestic animal for private purposes. [Ibid., 280, 281.] There cannot be the slightest doubt, says Robertson Smith, that the slaughter of a victim was originally among the acts which 'are illegal to an

Totem and Taboo

individual, and can only be justified when the whole clan shares the responsibility of the deed.[1] So far as I know, there is only one class of actions recognized by early nations to which this description applies, viz. actions which involve an invasion of the sanctity of the tribal blood. In fact, a life which no single tribesman is allowed to invade, and which can be sacrificed only by the consent and common action of the kin, stands on the same footing with the life of the fellow-tribesman.' The rule that every participant at the sacrificial meal must eat a share of the flesh of the victim has the same meaning as the provision that the execution of a guilty tribesman must be carried out by the tribe as a whole. [Ibid., 284–5.] In other words, the sacrificial animal was treated as a member of the tribe; the sacrificing community, the god and the sacrificial animal were of the same blood and members of one clan.[2]

Robertson Smith brings forward copious evidence for identifying the sacrificial animal with the primitive totem animal. In later antiquity there were two classes of sacrifice: one in which the victims were domestic animals of the kinds habitually used for eating, and the other extraordinary sacrifices of animals which were unclean and whose consumption was forbidden. Investigation shows that these unclean animals were sacred animals, that they were offered as sacrifices to the gods to whom they were sacred, that originally they were identical with the gods themselves, and that by means of the sacrifice the worshippers in some way laid stress upon their blood kinship with the animal and the god. [Ibid., 290–5.] But in still earlier times this distinction between ordinary and 'mystic' sacrifices disappears. Originally *all* [sacrificial] animals were sacred, their flesh was forbidden meat and might only be consumed on ceremonial occasions and with the participation of the whole clan. The slaughter of [such] an animal was equivalent to a shedding of the tribal blood and could occur subject only to the same precautions and the same insurances against incurring reproach. [Ibid., 312, 313.]

The domestication of animals and the introduction of cattle-breeding seems everywhere to have brought to an end the strict

[1] [This sentence is printed in spaced type by Freud.]
[2] [The last clause is in spaced type in the original.]

and unadulterated totemism of primæval days.[1] But such sacred character as remained to domestic animals under what had then become 'pastoral' religion is obvious enough to allow us to infer its original totemic nature. Even in late classical times ritual prescribed in many places that the sacrificial priest must take to flight after performing the sacrifice, as though to escape retribution. The idea that slaughtering oxen was a crime must at one time have prevailed generally in Greece. At the Athenian festival of Buphonia ['ox-murder'] a regular trial was instituted after the sacrifice, and all the participants were called as witnesses. At the end of it, it was agreed that the responsibility for the murder should be placed upon the knife; and this was accordingly cast into the sea. [Smith, 1894, 304.]

In spite of the ban protecting the lives of sacred animals in their quality of fellow-clansmen, a necessity arose for killing one of them from time to time in solemn communion and for dividing its flesh and blood among the members of the clan. The compelling motive for this deed reveals the deepest meaning of the nature of sacrifice. We have heard how in later times, whenever food is eaten in common, the participation in the same substance establishes a sacred bond between those who consume it when it has entered their bodies. In ancient times this result seems only to have been effected by participation in the substance of a *sacrosanct* victim. The holy mystery of sacrificial death 'is justified by the consideration that only in this way can the sacred cement be procured which creates or keeps alive a living bond of union between the worshippers and their god'.[2] (Ibid., 313.)

This bond is nothing else than the life of the sacrificial animal, which resides in its flesh and in its blood and is distributed among all the participants in the sacrificial meal. A notion of this kind lies at the root of all the blood covenants by which men made compacts with each other even at a late period of history. [Loc. cit.] This completely literal way of regarding blood-kinship as identity of substance makes it easy to under-

---

[1] 'The inference is that the domestication to which totemism inevitably leads (when there are any animals capable of domestication) is fatal to totemism.' (Jevons, 1902, 120.)

[2] [This sentence is printed in spaced type by Freud.]

stand the necessity for renewing it from time to time by the physical process of the sacrificial meal. [Ibid., 319.]

At this point I will interrupt my survey of Robertson Smith's line of thought and restate the gist of it in the most concise terms. With the establishment of the idea of private property sacrifice came to be looked upon as a gift to the deity, as a transference of property from men to the god. But this interpretation left unexplained all the peculiarities of the ritual of sacrifice. In the earliest times the sacrificial animal had itself been sacred and its life untouchable; it might only be killed if all the members of the clan participated in the deed and shared their guilt in the presence of the god, so that the sacred substance could be yielded up and consumed by the clansmen and thus ensure their identity with one another and with the deity. The sacrifice was a sacrament and the sacrificial animal was itself a member of the clan. It was in fact the ancient totem animal, the primitive god himself, by the killing and consuming of which the clansmen renewed and assured their likeness to the god.

From this analysis of the nature of sacrifice Robertson Smith draws the conclusion that the periodic killing and eating of the totem in times before the worship of anthropomorphic deities[1] had been an important element in totemic religion. [Ibid., 295.] The ceremonial of a totem meal of this kind is, he suggests, to be found in a description of a sacrifice of comparatively late date. St. Nilus records a sacrificial ritual current among the Bedouin of the Sinai Desert at the end of the fourth century A.D. The victim of the sacrifice, a camel, 'is bound upon a rude altar of stones piled together, and when the leader of the band has thrice led the worshippers round the altar in a solemn procession accompanied with chants, he inflicts the first wound . . . and in all haste drinks of the blood that gushes forth. Forthwith the whole company fall on the victim with their swords, hacking off pieces of the quivering flesh and devouring them raw with such wild haste, that in the short interval between the rise of the day star[2] which marked the hour for the service to begin, and the disappearance of its rays before the rising sun, the entire camel, body and bones, skin, blood and entrails, is wholly devoured.'

[1] [The last six words are in spaced type in the original.]
[2] To which the sacrifice was offered.

[Ibid., 338.] All the evidence goes to show that this barbaric ritual, which bears every sign of extreme antiquity, was no isolated instance but was everywhere the original form taken by totemic sacrifice, though later toned down in many different directions.

Many authorities have refused to attach importance to the concept of the totem meal, because it was not supported by any direct observation at the level of totemism. Robertson Smith himself pointed to instances in which the sacramental signi-ficance of the sacrifice seemed to be assured: for instance, the human sacrifices of the Aztecs, and others which recall the cir-cumstances of the totem meal—the sacrifice of bears by the Bear clan of the Ouataouak [Otawa] tribe in America and the bear feast of the Aino in Japan. [Ibid., 295 n.] These and similar cases have been reported in detail by Frazer in the Fifth Part of his great work (1912, 2 [Chaps. X, XIII, XIV]). An American Indian tribe in California, which worship a large bird of prey (a buzzard), kill it once a year at a solemn festival, after which it is mourned and its skin and feathers are preserved. [Ibid., **2**, 170.] The Zuni Indians of New Mexico behave in a similar way to their sacred turtles. [Ibid., **2**, 175.]

A feature has been observed in the *intichiuma* ceremonies of the Central Australian tribes which agrees admirably with Robertson Smith's conjectures. Each clan, when it is perform-ing magic for the multiplication of its totem (which it itself is normally prohibited from consuming), is obliged during the ceremony to eat a small portion of its own totem before making it accessible to the other clans. [Frazer, 1910, **1**, 110 ff.] Accord-ing to Frazer (ibid., **2**, 590) the clearest example of a sacra-mental consumption of an otherwise prohibited totem is to be found among the Bini of West Africa in connection with their funeral ceremonies.

Accordingly, I propose that we should adopt Robertson Smith's hypothesis that the sacramental killing and communal eating of the totem animal, whose consumption was forbidden on all other occasions, was an important feature of totemic religion.[1]

---

[1] I am not unaware of the objections to this theory of sacrifice which have been brought forward by various writers (such as Marillier [1898,

(5)

Let us call up the spectacle of a totem meal of the kind we have been discussing, amplified by a few probable features which we have not yet been able to consider. The clan is celebrating the ceremonial occasion by the cruel slaughter of its totem animal and is devouring it raw—blood, flesh and bones. The clansmen are there, dressed in the likeness of the totem and imitating it in sound and movement, as though they are seeking to stress their identity with it. Each man is conscious that he is performing an act forbidden to the individual and justifiable only through the participation of the whole clan; nor may anyone absent himself from the killing and the meal. When the deed is done, the slaughtered animal is lamented and bewailed. The mourning is obligatory, imposed by dread of a threatened retribution. As Robertson Smith (1894, 412) remarks of an analogous occasion, its chief purpose is to disclaim responsibility for the killing.

But the mourning is followed by demonstrations of festive rejoicing: every instinct is unfettered and there is licence for every kind of gratification. Here we have easy access to an understanding of the nature of festivals in general. A festival is a permitted, or rather an obligatory, excess, a solemn breach of a prohibition. It is not that men commit the excesses because they are feeling happy as a result of some injunction they have received. It is rather that excess is of the essence of a festival; the festive feeling is produced by the liberty to do what is as a rule prohibited.

What are we to make, though, of the prelude to this festive joy—the mourning over the death of the animal? If the clansmen rejoice over the killing of the totem—a normally forbidden act—why do they mourn over it as well?

As we have seen, the clansmen acquire sanctity by consuming the totem: they reinforce their identification with it and with one another. Their festive feelings and all that follows from them might well be explained by the fact that they have

204 ff.], Hubert and Mauss [1899, 30 ff.], etc.); but they have not diminished to any important extent the impression produced by Robertson Smith's hypothesis.

taken into themselves the sacred life of which the substance of the totem is the vehicle.

Psycho-analysis has revealed that the totem animal is in reality a substitute for the father; and this tallies with the contradictory fact that, though the killing of the animal is as a rule forbidden, yet its killing becomes a festive occasion—the fact that it is killed and yet mourned. The ambivalent emotional attitude, which to this day characterizes the father-complex in our children and which often persists into adult life, seems to extend to the totem animal in its capacity as substitute for the father.

If, now, we bring together the psycho-analytic translation of the totem with the fact of the totem meal and with Darwin's theories of the earliest state of human society, the possibility of a deeper understanding emerges—a glimpse of a hypothesis which may seem fantastic but which offers the advantage of establishing an unsuspected correlation between groups of phenomena that have hitherto been disconnected.

There is, of course, no place for the beginnings of totemism in Darwin's primal horde. All that we find there is a violent and jealous father who keeps all the females for himself and drives away his sons as they grow up. This earliest state of society has never been an object of observation. The most primitive kind of organization that we actually come across—and one that is in force to this day in certain tribes—consists of bands of males; these bands are composed of members with equal rights and are subject to the restrictions of the totemic system, including inheritance through the mother. Can this form of organization have developed out of the other one? and if so along what lines?

If we call the celebration of the totem meal to our help, we shall be able to find an answer. One day[1] the brothers who had been driven out came together, killed and devoured their father and so made an end of the patriarchal horde. United, they had the courage to do and succeeded in doing what would have been impossible for them individually. (Some cultural advance, perhaps, command over some new weapon, had given them a sense

[1] To avoid possible misunderstanding, I must ask the reader to take into account the final sentences of the following footnote as a corrective to this description.

Totem and Taboo

of superior strength.) Cannibal savages as they were, it goes without saying that they devoured their victim as well as killing him. The violent primal father had doubtless been the feared and envied model of each one of the company of brothers: and in the act of devouring him they accomplished their identification with him, and each one of them acquired a portion of his strength. The totem meal, which is perhaps mankind's earliest festival, would thus be a repetition and a commemoration of this memorable and criminal deed, which was the beginning of so many things—of social organization, of moral restrictions and of religion.[1]

[1] This hypothesis, which has such a monstrous air, of the tyrannical father being overwhelmed and killed by a combination of his exiled sons was also arrived at by Atkinson (1903, 220 f.) as a direct implication of the state of affairs in Darwin's primal horde: 'The patriarch had only one enemy whom he should dread . . . a youthful band of brothers living together in forced celibacy, or at most in polyandrous relation with some single female captive. A horde as yet weak in their impubescence they are, but they would, when strength was gained with time, inevitably wrench by combined attacks, renewed again and again, both wife and life from the paternal tyrant.' Atkinson, who incidentally passed his whole life in New Caledonia and had unusual opportunities for studying the natives, also pointed out that the conditions which Darwin assumed to prevail in the primal horde may easily be observed in herds of wild oxen and horses and regularly lead to the killing of the father of the herd. [Ibid., 222 f.] He further supposed that, after the father had been disposed of, the horde would be disintegrated by a bitter struggle between the victorious sons. Thus any new organization of society would be precluded: there would be 'an ever-recurring violent succession to the solitary paternal tyrant, by sons whose parricidal hands were so soon again clenched in fratricidal strife.' (Ibid., 228.) Atkinson, who had no psycho-analytic hints to help him and who was ignorant of Robertson Smith's studies, found a less violent transition from the primal horde to the next social stage, at which numbers of males live together in a peaceable community. He believed that through the intervention of maternal love the sons—to begin with only the youngest, but later others as well —were allowed to remain with the horde, and that in return for this toleration the sons acknowledged their father's sexual privilege by renouncing all claim to their mother and sisters. [Ibid., 231 ff.]

Such is the highly remarkable theory put forward by Atkinson. In its essential feature it is in agreement with my own; but its divergence results in its failing to effect a correlation with many other issues.

The lack of precision in what I have written in the text above, its abbreviation of the time factor and its compression of the whole subject-

The Return of Totemism in Childhood

In order that these latter consequences may seem plausible, leaving their premises on one side, we need only suppose that the tumultuous mob of brothers were filled with the same contradictory feelings which we can see at work in the ambivalent father-complexes of our children and of our neurotic patients. They hated their father, who presented such a formidable obstacle to their craving for power and their sexual desires; but they loved and admired him too. After they had got rid of him, had satisfied their hatred and had put into effect their wish to identify themselves with him, the affection which had all this time been pushed under was bound to make itself felt.[1] It did so in the form of remorse. A sense of guilt made its appearance, which in this instance coincided with the remorse felt by the whole group. The dead father became stronger than the living one had been—for events took the course we so often see them follow in human affairs to this day. What had up to then been prevented by his actual existence was thenceforward prohibited by the sons themselves, in accordance with the psychological procedure so familiar to us in psycho-analyses under the name of 'deferred obedience'. They revoked their deed by forbidding the killing of the totem, the substitute for their father; and they renounced its fruits by resigning their claim to the women who had now been set free. They thus created out of their filial sense of guilt the two fundamental taboos of totemism, which for that very reason inevitably corresponded to the two repressed wishes of the Œdipus complex. Whoever contravened those taboos became guilty of the only two crimes with which primitive society concerned itself.[2]

matter, may be attributed to the reserve necessitated by the nature of the topic. It would be as foolish to aim at exactitude in such questions as it would be unfair to insist upon certainty.

[1] This fresh emotional attitude must also have been assisted by the fact that the deed cannot have given complete satisfaction to those who did it. From one point of view it had been done in vain. Not one of the sons had in fact been able to put his original wish—of taking his father's place—into effect. And, as we know, failure is far more propitious for a moral reaction than satisfaction.

[2] 'Murder and incest, or offences of a like kind against the sacred laws of blood, are in primitive society the only crimes of which the community as such takes cognizance.' (Smith, 1894, 419.)

Totem and Taboo

The two taboos of totemism with which human morality has its beginning, are not on a par psychologically. The first of them, the law protecting the totem animal, is founded wholly on emotional motives: the father had actually been eliminated, and in no real sense could the deed be undone. But the second rule, the prohibition of incest, has a powerful practical basis as well. Sexual desires do not unite men but divide them. Though the brothers had banded together in order to overcome their father, they were all one another's rivals in regard to the women. Each of them would have wished, like his father, to have all the women to himself. The new organization would have collapsed in a struggle of all against all, for none of them was of such over-mastering strength as to be able to take on his father's part with success. Thus the brothers had no alternative, if they were to live together, but—not, perhaps, until they had passed through many dangerous crises—to institute the law against incest, by which they all alike renounced the women whom they desired and who had been their chief motive for despatching their father. In this way they rescued the organization which had made them strong—and which may have been based on homosexual feelings and acts, originating perhaps during the period of their expulsion from the horde. Here, too, may perhaps have been the germ of the institution of matriarchy, described by Bachofen [1861], which was in turn replaced by the patriarchal organization of the family.

On the other hand, the claim of totemism to be regarded as a first attempt at a religion is based on the first of these two taboos—that upon taking the life of the totem animal. The animal struck the sons as a natural and obvious substitute for their father; but the treatment of it which they found imposed on themselves expressed more than the need to exhibit their remorse. They could attempt, in their relation to this surrogate father, to allay their burning sense of guilt, to bring about a kind of reconciliation with their father. The totemic system was, as it were, a covenant with their father, in which he promised them everything that a childish imagination may expect from a father —protection, care and indulgence—while on their side they undertook to respect his life, that is to say, not to repeat the deed which had brought destruction on their real father.

Totemism, moreover, contained an attempt at self-justification: 'If our father had treated us in the way the totem does, we should never have felt tempted to kill him.' In this fashion totemism helped to smooth things over and to make it possible to forget the event to which it owed its origin.

Features were thus brought into existence which continued thenceforward to have a determining influence on the nature of religion. Totemic religion arose from the filial sense of guilt, in an attempt to allay that feeling and to appease the father by deferred obedience to him. All later religions are seen to be attempts at solving the same problem. They vary according to the stage of civilization at which they arise and according to the methods which they adopt; but all have the same end in view and are reactions to the same great event with which civilization began and which, since it occurred, has not allowed mankind a moment's rest.

There is another feature which was already present in totemism and which has been preserved unaltered in religion. The tension of ambivalence was evidently too great for any contrivance to be able to counteract it; or it is possible that psychological conditions in general are unfavourable to getting rid of these antithetical emotions. However that may be, we find that the ambivalence implicit in the father-complex persists in totemism and in religions generally. Totemic religion not only comprised expressions of remorse and attempts at atonement, it also served as a remembrance of the triumph over the father. Satisfaction over that triumph led to the institution of the memorial festival of the totem meal, in which the restrictions of deferred obedience no longer held. Thus it became a duty to repeat the crime of parricide again and again in the sacrifice of the totem animal, whenever, as a result of the changing conditions of life, the cherished fruit of the crime—appropriation of the paternal attributes—threatened to disappear. We shall not be surprised to find that the element of filial rebelliousness also emerges, in the *later* products of religion, often in the strangest disguises and transformations.

Hitherto we have followed the developments of the *affectionate* current of feeling towards the father, transformed into remorse, as we find them in religion and in moral ordinances (which are

145

not sharply distinguished in totemism). But we must not over-look the fact that it was in the main with the impulses that led to parricide that the victory lay. For a long time afterwards, the social fraternal feelings, which were the basis of the whole trans-formation, continued to exercise a profound influence on the development of society. They found expression in the sancti-fication of the blood tie, in the emphasis upon the solidarity of all life within the same clan. In thus guaranteeing one another's lives, the brothers were declaring that no one of them must be treated by another as their father was treated by them all jointly. They were precluding the possibility of a repetition of their father's fate. To the religiously based prohibition against killing the totem was now added the socially based prohibition against fratricide. It was not until long afterwards that the pro-hibition ceased to be limited to members of the clan and assumed the simple form: 'Thou shalt do no murder.' The patriarchal horde was replaced in the first instance by the fra-ternal clan, whose existence was assured by the blood tie. Society was now based on complicity in the common crime; religion was based on the sense of guilt and the remorse attach-ing to it; while morality was based partly on the exigencies of this society and partly on the penance demanded by the sense of guilt.

Thus psycho-analysis, in contradiction to the more recent views of the totemic system but in agreement with the earlier ones, requires us to assume that totemism and exogamy were intimately connected and had a simultaneous origin.

(6)

A great number of powerful motives restrain me from any attempt at picturing the further development of religions from their origin in totemism to their condition to-day. I will only follow two threads whose course I can trace with especial clarity as they run through the pattern: the theme of the totemic sacri-fice and the relation of son to father.[1]

[1] Cf. the discussion by C. G. Jung (1912), which is governed by views differing in certain respects from mine.

The Return of Totemism in Childhood

Robertson Smith has shown us that the ancient totem meal recurs in the original form of sacrifice. The meaning of the act is the same: sanctification through participation in a common meal. The sense of guilt, which can only be allayed by the solidarity of all the participants, also persists. What is new is the clan deity, in whose supposed presence the sacrifice is performed, who participates in the meal as though he were a clansman, and with whom those who consume the meal become identified. How does the god come to be in a situation to which he was originally a stranger?

The answer might be that in the meantime the concept of God had emerged—from some unknown source—and had taken control of the whole of religious life; and that, like everything else that was to survive, the totem meal had been obliged to find a point of contact with the new system. The psychoanalysis of individual human beings, however, teaches us with quite special insistence that the god of each of them is formed in the likeness of his father, that his personal relation to God depends on his relation to his father in the flesh and oscillates and changes along with that relation, and that at bottom God is nothing other than an exalted father. As in the case of totemism, psycho-analysis recommends us to have faith in the believers who call God their father, just as the totem was called the tribal ancestor. If psycho-analysis deserves any attention, then—without prejudice to any other sources or meanings of the concept of God, upon which psycho-analysis can throw no light—the paternal element in that concept must be a most important one. But in that case the father is represented twice over in the situation of primitive sacrifice: once as God and once as the totemic animal victim. And, even granting the restricted number of explanations open to psycho-analysis, one must ask whether this is possible and what sense it can have.

We know that there are a multiplicity of relations between the god and the sacred animal (the totem or the sacrificial victim). (1) Each god usually has an animal (and quite often several animals) sacred to him. (2) In the case of certain specially sacred sacrifices—'mystic' sacrifices—the victim was precisely the animal sacred to the god (Smith, 1894 [290]). (3) The god was often worshipped in the shape of an animal (or,

147

to look at it in another way, animals were worshipped as gods) long after the age of totemism. (4) In myths the god often transforms himself into an animal, and frequently into the animal that is sacred to him.

It therefore seems plausible to suppose that the god himself was the totem animal, and that he developed out of it at a later stage of religious feeling. But we are relieved from the necessity for further discussion by the consideration that the totem is nothing other than a surrogate of the father. Thus, while the totem may be the *first* form of father-surrogate, the god will be a later one, in which the father has regained his human shape. A new creation such as this, derived from what constitutes the root of every form of religion—a longing for the father—might occur if in the process of time some fundamental change had taken place in man's relation to the father, and perhaps, too, in his relation to animals.

Signs of the occurrence of changes of this kind may easily be seen, even if we leave on one side the beginning of a mental estrangement from animals and the disrupting of totemism owing to domestication. (See above, p. 136 f.) There was one factor in the state of affairs produced by the elimination of the father which was bound in the course of time to cause an enormous increase in the longing felt for him. Each single one of the brothers who had banded together for the purpose of killing their father was inspired by a wish to become like him and had given expression to it by incorporating parts of their father's surrogate in the totem meal. But, in consequence of the pressure exercised upon each participant by the fraternal clan as a whole, that wish could not be fulfilled. For the future no one could or might ever again attain the father's supreme power, even though that was what all of them had striven for. Thus after a long lapse of time their bitterness against their father, which had driven them to their deed, grew less, and their longing for him increased; and it became possible for an ideal to emerge which embodied the unlimited power of the primal father against whom they had once fought as well as their readiness to submit to him. As a result of decisive cultural changes, the original democratic equality that had prevailed among all the individual clansmen became untenable; and there developed at the same time an inclination, based on veneration felt for particular human individuals, to revive the ancient paternal ideal by creating gods. The notion of a man becoming a god or of a god dying strikes us to-day as shockingly presumptuous; but even in classical antiquity there was nothing revolting in it.[1] The elevation of the father who had once been murdered into a god from whom the clan claimed descent was a far more serious attempt at atonement than had been the ancient covenant with the totem.

I cannot suggest at what point in this process of development a place is to be found for the great mother-goddesses, who may perhaps in general have preceded the father-gods. It seems certain, however, that the change in attitude to the father was not restricted to the sphere of religion but that it extended in a consistent manner to that other side of human life which had been affected by the father's removal—to social organization. With the introduction of father-deities a fatherless society gradually changed into one organized on a patriarchal basis. The family was a restoration of the former primal horde and it gave back to fathers a large portion of their former rights. There were once more fathers, but the social achievements of the fraternal clan had not been abandoned; and the gulf between the new fathers of a family and the unrestricted primal father of the horde was wide enough to guarantee the continuance of the religious craving, the persistence of an unappeased longing for the father.

We see, then, that in the scene of sacrifice before the god of the clan the father *is* in fact represented twice over—as the god and as the totemic animal victim. But in our attempts at understanding this situation we must beware of interpretations which seek to translate it in a two-dimensional fashion as though it were an allegory, and which in so doing forget its historical stratification. The two-fold presence of the father corresponds to the two chronologically successive meanings of the scene. The

---

[1] 'To us moderns, for whom the breach which divides the human and the divine has deepened into an impassable gulf, such mimicry may appear impious, but it was otherwise with the ancients. To their thinking gods and men were akin, for many families traced their descent from a divinity, and the deification of a man probably seemed as little extraordinary to them as the canonization of a saint seems to a modern Catholic.' (Frazer, 1911*a*, **2**, 177 f.)

ambivalent attitude towards the father has found a plastic expression in it, and so, too, has the victory of the son's affectionate emotions over his hostile ones. The scene of the father's vanquishment, of his greatest defeat, has become the stuff for the representation of his supreme triumph. The importance which is everywhere, without exception, ascribed to sacrifice lies in the fact that it offers satisfaction to the father for the outrage inflicted on him in the same act in which that deed is commemorated.

As time went on, the animal lost its sacred character and the sacrifice lost its connection with the totem feast; it became a simple offering to the deity, an act of renunciation in favour of the god. God Himself had become so far exalted above mankind that He could only be approached through an intermediary—the priest. At the same time divine kings made their appearance in the social structure and introduced the patriarchal system into the state. It must be confessed that the revenge taken by the deposed and restored father was a harsh one: the dominance of authority was at its climax. The subjugated sons made use of the new situation in order to unburden themselves still further of their sense of guilt. They were no longer in any way responsible for the sacrifice as it now was. It was God Himself who demanded it and regulated it. This is the phase in which we find myths showing the god himself killing the animal which is sacred to him and which is in fact himself. Here we have the most extreme denial of the great crime which was the beginning of society and of the sense of guilt. But there is a second meaning to this last picture of sacrifice which is unmistakable. It expresses satisfaction at the earlier father-surrogate having been abandoned in favour of the superior concept of God. At this point the psycho-analytic interpretation of the scene coincides approximately with the allegorical, surface translation of it, which represents the god as overcoming the animal side of his own nature.[1]

[1] It is generally agreed that when, in mythologies, one generation of gods is overcome by another, what is denoted is the historical replacement of one religious system by a new one, whether as a result of foreign conquest or of psychological development. In the latter case myth approximates to what Silberer [1909] has described as 'functional

Nevertheless it would be a mistake to suppose that the hostile impulses inherent in the father-complex were completely silenced during this period of revived paternal authority. On the contrary, the first phases of the dominance of the two new father-surrogates—gods and kings—show the most energetic signs of the ambivalence that remains a characteristic of religion.

In his great work, *The Golden Bough*, Frazer [1911*a*, 2, Chap. XVIII] puts forward the view that the earliest kings of the Latin tribes were foreigners who played the part of a god and were solemnly executed at a particular festival. The annual sacrifice (or, as a variant, self-sacrifice) of a god seems to have been an essential element in the Semitic religions. The ceremonials of human sacrifice, performed in the most different parts of the inhabited globe, leave very little doubt that the victims met their end as representatives of the deity; and these sacrificial rites can be traced into late times, with an inanimate effigy or puppet taking the place of the living human being. The theanthropic sacrifice of the god, into which it is unfortunately impossible for me to enter here as fully as into animal sacrifice, throws a searching retrospective light upon the meaning of the older forms of sacrifice. [Smith, 1894, 410 f.] It confesses, with a frankness that could hardly be excelled, to the fact that the object of the act of sacrifice has always been the same—namely what is now worshipped as God, that is to say, the father. The problem of the relation between animal and human sacrifice thus admits of a simple solution. The original animal sacrifice was already a substitute for a human sacrifice—for the ceremonial killing of the father; so that, when the father-surrogate once more resumed its human shape, the animal sacrifice too could be changed back into a human sacrifice.

The memory of the first great act of sacrifice thus proved indestructible, in spite of every effort to forget it; and at the very point at which men sought to be at the farthest distance from the motives that led to it, its undistorted reproduction emerged

phenomena'. [Cf. Freud, 1900, English translation, 1932, 464 ff.] The view maintained by Jung (1912) that the god who kills the animal is a libidinal symbol implies a concept of libido other than that which has hitherto been employed and seems to me questionable from every point of view.

in the form of the sacrifice of the god. I need not enlarge here upon the developments of religious thought which, in the shape of rationalizations, made this recurrence possible. Robertson Smith, who had no thought of our derivation of sacrifice from the great event in human prehistory, states that the ceremonies at the festivals in which the ancient Semites celebrated the death of a deity 'were currently interpreted as the commemoration of a mythical tragedy' [ibid., 413]. 'The mourning', he declares, 'is not a spontaneous expression of sympathy with the divine tragedy, but obligatory and enforced by fear of supernatural anger. And a chief object of the mourners is to disclaim responsibility for the god's death—a point which has already come before us in connection with theanthropic sacrifices, such as the "ox-murder at Athens".' (Ibid., 412.) It seems most probable that these 'current interpretations' were correct and that the feelings of the celebrants were fully explained by the underlying situation.

Let us assume it to be a fact, then, that in the course of the later development of religions the two driving factors, the son's sense of guilt and the son's rebelliousness, never became extinct. Whatever attempt was made at solving the religious problem, whatever kind of reconciliation was effected between these two opposing mental forces, sooner or later broke down, under the combined influence, no doubt, of historical events, cultural changes and internal psychical modifications.

The son's efforts to put himself in the place of the father-god became ever more obvious. The introduction of agriculture increased the son's importance in the patriarchal family. He ventured upon new demonstrations of his incestuous libido, which found symbolic satisfaction in his cultivation of Mother Earth. Divine figures such as Attis, Adonis and Tammuz emerged, spirits of vegetation and at the same time youthful divinities enjoying the favours of mother goddesses and committing incest with their mother in defiance of their father. But the sense of guilt, which was not allayed by these creations, found expression in myths which granted only short lives to these youthful favourites of the mother-goddesses and decreed their punishment by emasculation or by the wrath of the father in the form of an animal. Adonis was killed by a wild boar, the sacred animal of

152

Aphrodite; Attis, beloved of Cybele, perished by castration.[1]
The mourning for these gods and the rejoicings over their resur-
rection passed over into the ritual of another son-deity who was
destined to lasting success.

When Christianity first penetrated into the ancient world it
met with competition from the religion of Mithras and for a
time it was doubtful which of the two deities would gain the
victory. In spite of the halo of light surrounding his form, the
youthful Persian god remains obscure to us. We may perhaps
infer from the sculptures of Mithras slaying a bull that he represented a son who was alone in sacrificing his father and thus redeemed his brothers from their burden of complicity in the
deed. There was an alternative method of allaying their guilt
and this was first adopted by Christ. He sacrificed his own life
and so redeemed the company of brothers from original sin.

The doctrine of original sin was of Orphic origin. It formed a
part of the mysteries, and spread from them to the schools of
philosophy of ancient Greece. (Reinach, 1905-12, 2, 75 ff.)
Mankind, it was said, were descended from the Titans, who had
killed the young Dionysus-Zagreus and had torn him to pieces.
The burden of this crime weighed on them. A fragment of
Anaximander relates how the unity of the world was broken by
a primæval sin,[2] and that whatever issued from it must bear the

[1] Fear of castration plays an extremely large part, in the case of the
youthful neurotics whom we come across, as an interference in their
relations with their father. The illuminating instance reported by Ferenczi (1913a) has shown us how a little boy took as his totem the beast
that had snapped at his little penis. [See page 130 f.] When our children
come to hear of ritual circumcision, they equate it with castration. The
parallel in social psychology to this reaction by children has not yet been
worked out, so far as I am aware. In primæval times and in primitive
races, where circumcision is so frequent, it is performed at the age of
initiation into manhood and it is at that age that its significance is to be
found; it was only as a secondary development that it was shifted back
to the early years of life. It is of very great interest to find that among
primitive peoples circumcision is combined with cutting the hair and
knocking out teeth or is replaced by them, and that our children, who
cannot possibly have any knowledge of this, in fact treat these two operations, in the anxiety with which they react to them, as equivalents of
castration.

[2] 'Une sorte de péché proethnique' (Reinach, 1905-12, 2, 76).

punishment. The tumultuous mobbing, the killing and the tearing in pieces by the Titans reminds us clearly enough of the totemic sacrifice described by St. Nilus [ibid., 2, 93]—as, for the matter of that, do many other ancient myths, including, for instance, that of the death of Orpheus himself. Nevertheless, there is a disturbing difference in the fact of the murder having been committed on a *youthful* god.

There can be no doubt that in the Christian myth the original sin was one against God the Father. If, however, Christ redeemed mankind from the burden of original sin by the sacrifice of his own life, we are driven to conclude that the sin was a murder. The law of talion, which is so deeply rooted in human feelings, lays it down that a murder can only be expiated by the sacrifice of another life: self-sacrifice points back to blood-guilt.[1] And if this sacrifice of a life brought about atonement with God the Father, the crime to be expiated can only have been the murder of the father.

In the Christian doctrine, therefore, men were acknowledging in the most undisguised manner the guilty primæval deed, since they found the fullest atonement for it in the sacrifice of this one son. Atonement with the father was all the more complete since the sacrifice was accompanied by a total renunciation of the women on whose account the rebellion against the father was started. But at that point the inexorable psychological law of ambivalence stepped in. The very deed in which the son offered the greatest possible atonement to the father brought him at the same time to the attainment of his wishes *against* the father. He himself became God, beside, or, more correctly, in place of, the father. A son-religion displaced the father-religion. As a sign of this substitution the ancient totem meal was revived in the form of communion, in which the company of brothers consumed the flesh and blood of the son—no longer the father—obtained sanctity thereby and identified themselves with him. Thus we can trace through the ages the identity of the totem meal with animal sacrifice, with theanthropic human sacrifice and with the Christian Eucharist, and we can recognize in all these rituals the effect of the crime by which men were so deeply

[1] We find that impulses to suicide in a neurotic turn out regularly to be self-punishments for wishes for someone else's death.

weighed down but of which they must none the less feel so proud. The Christian communion, however, is essentially a fresh elimination of the father, a repetition of the guilty deed. We can see the full justice of Frazer's pronouncement that 'the Christian communion has absorbed within itself a sacrament which is doubtless far older than Christianity'.[1]

(7)

An event such as the elimination of the primal father by the company of his sons must inevitably have left ineradicable traces in the history of humanity; and the less it itself was recollected, the more numerous must have been the substitutes to which it gave rise.[2] I shall resist the temptation of pointing out these traces in mythology, where they are not hard to find, and shall turn in another direction and take up a suggestion made by Salomon Reinach in a most instructive essay on the death of Orpheus.[3]

In the history of Greek art we come upon a situation which shows striking resemblances to the scene of the totem meal as identified by Robertson Smith, and not less profound differences from it. I have in mind the situation of the most ancient Greek tragedy. A company of individuals, named and dressed alike, surrounded a single figure, all hanging upon his words and deeds: they were the Chorus and the impersonator of the Hero. He was originally the only actor. Later, a second and third actor were added, to play as counterpart to the Hero and as characters split off from him; but the character of the Hero

---

[1] Frazer (1912, **2**, 51). No one familiar with the literature of the subject will imagine that the derivation of Christian communion from the totem meal is an idea originating from the author of the present essay.

[2] In Ariel's words from *The Tempest*:
'Full fathom five thy father lies;
Of his bones are coral made;
Those are pearls that were his eyes:
Nothing of him that doth fade,
But doth suffer a sea-change
Into something rich and strange.'

[3] 'La mort d'Orphée', contained in the volume which I have so often quoted (1905–12, **2**, 100 ff.).

himself and his relation to the Chorus remained unaltered. The Hero of tragedy must suffer; to this day that remains the essence of a tragedy. He had to bear the burden of what was known as 'tragic guilt'; the basis of that guilt is not always easy to find, for in the light of our everyday life it is often no guilt at all. As a rule it lay in rebellion against some divine or human authority; and the Chorus accompanied the Hero with feelings of sympathy, sought to hold him back, to warn him and to sober him, and mourned over him when he had met with what was felt as the merited punishment for his rash undertaking.

But why had the Hero of tragedy to suffer? and what was the meaning of his 'tragic guilt'? I will cut the discussion short and give a quick reply. He had to suffer because he was the primal father, the Hero of the great primæval tragedy which was being re-enacted with a tendentious twist; and the tragic guilt was the guilt which he had to take on himself in order to relieve the Chorus from theirs. The scene upon the stage was derived from the historical scene through a process of systematic distortion—one might even say, as the product of a refined hypocrisy. In the remote reality it had actually been the members of the Chorus who caused the Hero's suffering; now, however, they exhausted themselves with sympathy and regret and it was the Hero himself who was responsible for his own sufferings. The crime which was thrown on to his shoulders, presumptuousness and rebelliousness against a great authority, was precisely the crime for which the members of the Chorus, the company of brothers, were responsible. Thus the tragic Hero became, though it might be against his will, the redeemer of the Chorus.

In Greek tragedy the special subject-matter of the performance was the sufferings of the divine goat, Dionysus, and the lamentation of the goats who were his followers and who identified themselves with him. That being so, it is easy to understand how drama, which had become extinct, was kindled into fresh life in the Middle Ages around the Passion of Christ.

At the conclusion, then, of this exceedingly condensed inquiry, I should like to insist that its outcome shows that the beginnings of religion, morals, society and art converge in the Œdipus complex. This is in complete agreement with the psycho-analytic finding that the same complex constitutes the nucleus of all neuroses, so far as our present knowledge goes. It seems to me a most surprising discovery that the problems of social psychology, too, should prove soluble on the basis of one single concrete point—man's relation to his father. It is even possible that yet another psychological problem belongs in this same connection. I have often had occasion to point out that emotional ambivalence in the proper sense of the term—that is, the simultaneous existence of love and hate towards the same object—lies at the root of many important cultural institutions. We know nothing of the origin of this ambivalence. One possible assumption is that it is a fundamental phenomenon of our emotional life. But it seems to me quite worth considering another possibility, namely that originally it formed no part of our emotional life but was acquired by the human race in connection with their father-complex,[1] precisely where the psycho-analytic examination of modern individuals still finds it revealed at its strongest.[2]

Before I bring my remarks to a close, however, I must find room to point out that, though my arguments have led to a high degree of convergence upon a single comprehensive nexus of ideas, this fact cannot blind us to the uncertainties of my premises or the difficulties involved in my conclusions. I will only mention two of the latter which may have forced themselves on the notice of a number of my readers.

No one can have failed to observe, in the first place, that I have taken as the basis of my whole position the existence of a collective mind, in which mental processes occur just as they do in the mind of an individual. In particular, I have supposed

[1] Or, more correctly, their parental complex.

[2] Since I am used to being misunderstood, I think it worth while to insist explicitly that the derivations which I have proposed in these pages do not in the least overlook the complexity of the phenomena under review. All that they claim is to have added a new factor to the sources, known or still unknown, of religion, morality and society—a factor based on a consideration of the implications of psycho-analysis. I must leave to others the task of synthesizing the explanation into a unity. It does, however, follow from the nature of the new contribution that it could not play any other than a central part in such a synthesis, even though powerful emotional resistances might have to be overcome before its great importance was recognized.

that the sense of guilt for an action has persisted for many thousands of years and has remained operative in generations which can have had no knowledge of that action. I have supposed that an emotional process, such as might have developed in generations of sons who were ill-treated by their father, has extended to new generations which were exempt from such treatment for the very reason that their father had been eliminated. It must be admitted that these are grave difficulties; and any explanation that could avoid presumptions of such a kind would seem to be preferable.

Further reflection, however, will show that I am not alone in the responsibility for this bold procedure. Without the assumption of a collective mind, which makes it possible to neglect the interruptions of mental acts caused by the extinction of the individual, social psychology in general cannot exist. Unless psychical processes were continued from one generation to another, if each generation were obliged to acquire its attitude to life anew, there would be no progress in this field and next to no development. This gives rise to two further questions: how much can we attribute to psychical continuity in the sequence of generations? and what are the ways and means employed by one generation in order to hand on its mental states to the next one? I shall not pretend that these problems are sufficiently explained or that direct communication and tradition—which are the first things that occur to one—are enough to account for the process. Social psychology shows very little interest, on the whole, in the manner in which the required continuity in the mental life of successive generations is established. A part of the problem seems to be met by the inheritance of psychical dispositions which, however, need to be given some sort of impetus in the life of the individual before they can be roused into actual operation. This may be the meaning of the poet's words:

'Was du ererbt von deinen Vätern hast,
Erwirb es, um es zu besitzen.'[1]

The problem would seem even more difficult if we had to admit

[1] [Goethe, *Faust*, Part I: 'What thou hast inherited from thy fathers, acquire it to make it thine.']

158

that mental impulses could be so completely suppressed as to leave no trace whatever behind them. But that is not the case. Even the most ruthless suppression must leave room for distorted surrogate impulses and for reactions resulting from them. If so, however, we may safely assume that no generation is able to conceal any of its more important mental processes from its successor. For psycho-analysis has shown us that everyone possesses in his unconscious mental activity an apparatus which enables him to interpret other people's reactions, that is, to undo the distortions which other people have imposed on the expression of their feelings. An unconscious understanding such as this of all the customs, ceremonies and dogmas left behind by the original relation to the father may have made it possible for later generations to take over their heritage of emotion.

Another difficulty might actually be brought forward from psycho-analytic quarters. The earliest moral precepts and restrictions in primitive society have been explained by us as reactions to a deed which gave those who performed it the concept of 'crime'. They felt remorse for the deed and decided that it should never be repeated and that its performance should bring no advantage. This creative sense of guilt still persists among us. We find it operating in an asocial manner in neurotics, and producing new moral precepts and persistent restrictions, as an atonement for crimes that have been committed and as a precaution against the committing of new ones.[1] If, however, we inquire among these neurotics to discover what were the deeds which provoked these reactions, we shall be disappointed. We find no deeds, but only impulses and emotions, set upon evil ends but held back from their achievement. What lie behind the sense of guilt of neurotics are always *psychical* realities and never *factual* ones. What characterizes neurotics is the fact that they prefer psychical to factual reality and react just as seriously to thoughts as normal persons do to realities.

May not the same have been true of primitive men? We are justified in believing that, as one of the phenomena of their narcissistic organization, they overvalued their psychical acts to an extraordinary degree.[2] Accordingly the mere hostile *impulse*

[1] Cf. the essay on taboo, the second in this volume [p. 67 ff.].
[2] Cf. the third essay in this volume [p. 85].

against the father, the mere existence of a wishful *phantasy* of killing and devouring him, would have been enough to produce the moral reaction that created totemism and taboo. In this way we should avoid the necessity for deriving the origin of our cultural legacy, of which we justly feel so proud, from a hideous crime, revolting to all our feelings. No damage would thus be done to the causal chain stretching from the beginning to the present day, for psychical reality would be strong enough to bear the weight of these consequences. To this it may be objected that an alteration in the form of society from a patriarchal horde to a fraternal clan did actually take place. This is a powerful argument, but not a conclusive one. The alteration might have been effected in a less violent fashion and none the less have been capable of determining the appearance of the moral reaction. So long as the pressure exercised by the primal father could be felt, the hostile feelings towards him were justified, and remorse on their account would have to await a later day. And if it is further argued that everything derived from the ambivalent relation to the father—taboo and the sacrificial ordinance—is characterized by the deepest seriousness and the most complete reality, this further objection carries just as little weight. For the ceremonials and inhibitions of obsessional neurotics show these same characteristics and are nevertheless derived only from psychical reality—from intentions and not from their execution. We must avoid transplanting a contempt for what is merely thought or wished from our commonplace world, with its wealth of material values, into the world of primitive men and neurotics, of which the wealth lies only within themselves.

Here we are faced by a decision which is indeed no easy one. First, however, it must be confessed that the distinction, which may seem fundamental to other people, does not in our judgment affect the heart of the matter. If wishes and impulses have the full value of facts for primitive men, it is our business to give their attitude our understanding attention instead of correcting it in accordance with our own standards. Let us, then, examine more closely the case of neurosis—comparison with which led us into our present uncertainty. It is not accurate to say that obsessional neurotics, weighed down under the burden of an excessive morality, are defending themselves only against *psy-*

chical reality and are punishing themselves for impulses which were merely *felt*. *Historical* reality has a share in the matter as well. In their childhood they had these evil impulses pure and simple, and turned them into acts so far as the impotence of childhood allowed. Each of these excessively virtuous individuals passed through an evil period in his infancy—a phase of perversion which was the forerunner and precondition of the later period of excessive morality. The analogy between primitive men and neurotics will therefore be far more fully established if we suppose that in the former instance, too, psychical reality—as to the form taken by which we are in no doubt—coincided at the beginning with factual reality: that primitive men actually *did* what all the evidence shows that they intended to do.

Nor must we let ourselves be influenced too far in our judgment of primitive men by the analogy of neurotics. There are distinctions, too, which must be borne in mind. It is no doubt true that the sharp contrast that *we* make between thinking and doing is absent in both of them. But neurotics are above all *inhibited* in their actions: with them the thought is a complete substitute for the deed. Primitive men, on the other hand, are *uninhibited:* thought passes directly into action. With them it is rather the deed that is a substitute for the thought. And that is why, without laying claim to any finality of judgment, I think that in the case before us it may safely be assumed that 'in the beginning was the Deed'.[1]

[1] ['*Im Anfang war die Tat*' (Goethe, *Faust*, Part I).]

List of Works
Referred to in the Text

[Titles of books and periodicals are in italics; titles of papers are in inverted commas. Abbreviations are in accordance with the *World List of Scientific Periodicals* (Oxford, 1934). Numerals in thick type refer to volumes; ordinary numerals refer to pages. '*Trans.*' before an entry indicates that any reference in the text is not to the original but to an English translation. *G.S.* =Freud, *Gesammelte Schriften* (12 vols.), Vienna, 1924–34. *G.W.* =Freud, *Gesammelte Werke* (18 vols.), London, 1940–. *C.P.* =Freud, *Collected Papers* (5 vols.), London, 1924–50.]

ABRAHAM, K. (1912). 'Über die determinierende Kraft des Namens', *Int. Z. Psychoanal.*, **2**, 133.
— (1914). 'Über Einschränkungen und Umwandlungen der Schaulust bei den Psychoneurotikern', *Jb. Psychoanal.*, **6**, 25.
(*Trans.*: 'Restrictions and Transformations of Scopophilia in Psycho-Neurotics', *Selected Papers*, 1927, 169.)
— (1927). *Selected Papers*, London.
ATKINSON, J. J. (1903). *Primal Law*, London. (Included in LANG, A., *Social Origins*.)
AVEBURY, Lord. *See* LUBBOCK, J.
BACHOFEN, J. J. (1861). *Das Mutterrecht*, Stuttgart.
BASTIAN, A. (1874–5). *Die deutsche Expedition an der Loango-Küste* (2 vols.), Jena.
BATCHELOR, J. (1901). *The Ainu and their Folk-Lore*, London.
BLUMENTRITT, F. (1891). 'Über die Eingeborenen der Insel Palawan', *Globus*, **59**, 181.
BOAS, F. (1888). 'The Central Eskimo', *Sixth Ann. Rep. Bur. Amer. Ethn.*, 399.
— (1890). 'Second General Report on the Indians of British Columbia', *Report of Sixtieth Meeting of the British Association*, 562.
BROWN, W. (1845). *New Zealand and its Aborigines*, London.
CAMERON, A. L. P. (1885). 'Notes on some Tribes of New South Wales', *J. anthrop. Inst.*, **14**, 344.

Bibliography

CODRINGTON, R. H. (1891). *The Melanesians*, Oxford.

CRAWLEY, E. (1902). *The Mystic Rose*, London.

DARWIN, C. (1871). *The Descent of Man* (2 vols.), London.

(1875). *The Variation of Animals and Plants under Domestication* (2 vols.), 2nd ed., London.

DOBRIZHOFFER, M. (1784). *Historia de Abiponibus* (3 vols.), Vienna.

DORSEY, J. O. (1884). 'An Account of the War Customs of the Osages', *Amer. Nat.*, **18**, 113.

DURKHEIM, E. (1898). 'La prohibition de l'inceste et ses origines', *Année sociolog.*, **1**, 1.

(1902). 'Sur le totémisme', *Année sociolog.*, **5**, 82.

(1905). 'Sur l'organisation matrimoniale des sociétés australiennes', *Année sociolog.*, **8**, 118.

(1912). *Les formes élémentaires de la vie religieuse: Le système totémique en Australie*, Paris.

EDER, M. D. (1913). 'Augenträume', *Int. Z. Psychoanal.* **1**, 157.

ELLIS, HAVELOCK (1914). *Sexual Selection in Man* (*Studies in the Psychology of Sex*, IV), Philadelphia.

ELLIS, W. (1832–6). *Polynesian Researches*, 2nd ed. (4 vols.), London.

Encyclopaedia Britannica (1910–11). Eleventh Edition, Cambridge.

FERENCZI, S. (1913a). 'Ein kleiner Hahnemann', *Int. Z. Psychoanal.*, **1**, 240.

(*Trans.*: 'A Little Chanticleer', *Contributions to Psycho-Analysis*, 1916, 240.)

(1913b). 'Zur Augensymbolik', *Int. Z. Psychoanal.*, **1**, 161.

(*Trans.*: 'On Eye Symbolism', *Contributions to Psycho-Analysis*, 1916, 270.)

(1916). *Contributions to Psycho-Analysis*, Boston. [Later title-page: *Sex in Psycho-Analysis*.]

FISON, L. (1885). 'The Nanga', *J. anthrop. Inst.*, **14**, 14.

FISON, L., and HOWITT, A. W. (1880). *Kamilaroi and Kurnai*, Melbourne.

FRASER, J. (1892). *The Aborigines of New South Wales*, Sydney.

FRAZER, J. G. (1910). *Totemism and Exogamy* (4 vols.), London.

(1911a). *The Magic Art* (2 vols.) (*The Golden Bough*, 3rd ed., Part I), London.

(1911b). *Taboo and the Perils of the Soul* (*The Golden Bough*, 3rd ed., Part II), London.

(1912). *Spirits of the Corn and of the Wild* (2 vols.) (*The Golden Bough*, 3rd ed., Part V), London.

(1914). *Adonis, Attis, Osiris*, 3rd ed. (2 vols.) (*The Golden Bough*, 3rd ed., Part IV), London.

Totem and Taboo

FREUD, S. (1900). *Die Traumdeutung*, Vienna. (*G.S.*, 2–3; *G.W.*, 2–3.)
(*Trans.*: *The Interpretation of Dreams*, revised ed., London, 1932.)
(1905*a*). *Drei Abhandlungen zur Sexualtheorie*, Vienna. (*G.S.*, 5, 1: *G.W.*, 5, 29)
(*Trans.*: *Three Essays on the Theory of Sexuality*, London, 1949.)
(1905*b*). *Der Witz und seine Beziehung zum Unbewussten*, Vienna. (*G.S.*, 9; *G.W.*, 6.)
(*Trans.*: *Wit and its Relation to the Unconscious*, London, 1922.)
(1909*a*). 'Analyse der Phobie eines fünfjährigen Knaben', *G.S.*, 8, 127; *G.W.*, 7, 243.
(*Trans.*: 'Analysis of a Phobia in a Five-Year-Old Boy', *C.P.*, 3, 149.)
(1909*b*). 'Bemerkungen über einen Fall von Zwangsneurose', *G.S.*, 8, 267; *G.W.*, 7, 381.
(*Trans.*: 'Notes upon a Case of Obsessional Neurosis', *C.P.*, 3, 293.)
(1910). ' "Über den Gegensinn der Urworte" ', *G.S.*, 10, 221; *G.W.*, 8, 214.
(*Trans.*: ' "The Antithetical Sense of Primal Words" ', *C.P.*, 4, 184.)
(1911*a*). 'Formulierungen über die zwei Principien des psychischen Geschehens', *G.S.*, 5, 409; *G.W.*, 8, 214.
(*Trans.*: 'Formulations regarding the Two Principles in Mental Functioning', *C.P.*, 4, 13.)
(1911*b*). 'Psychoanalytische Bemerkungen über einen autobiographisch beschriebenen Fall von Paranoia', *G.S.*, 8, 353; *G.W.*, 8, 240.
(*Trans.*: 'Psycho-Analytic Notes upon an Autobiographical Account of a Case of Paranoia', *C.P.*, 3, 387.)
(1912). 'Einige Bemerkungen über den Begriff des Unbewussten in der Psychoanalyse', *G.S.*, 5, 433; *G.W.*, 8, 430.
(*Trans.*: 'A Note on the Unconscious in Psycho-Analysis', *C.P.*, 4, 22.)
(1919). 'Das Unheimliche', *G.S.*, 10, 369; *G.W.*, 12, 236.
(*Trans.*: 'The Uncanny', *C.P.*, 4, 368.)
(1933). *Neue Folge der Vorlesungen zur Einführung in die Psychoanalyse*, Vienna. (*G.S.*, 12, 149; *G.W.*, 15, 1.)
(*Trans.*: *New Introductory Lectures on Psycho-Analysis*, London, 1933.)
GOLDENWEISER, A. (1910). 'Totemism, an Analytical Study', *J. Am. Folk-Lore*, 23, 179.
GRAMBERG, J. S. G. (1872). 'Eene maand in de binnenlanden van Timor', *Verh. batavia. Genoot.*, 36, 161.

Bibliography

Guis, Le Père J. (1902). 'Les Canaques', *Missions Catholiques*, **34**, 208.

Haddon, A. C. (1902). 'Presidential Address to the Anthropological Section', *Report of Seventy-Second Meeting of the British Association*, 738.

Haeberlin, P. (1912). 'Sexualgespenster', *Sexualprobleme*, February.

Howitt, A. W. (1904). *The Native Tribes of South-East Australia*, London.

Hubert, H., and Mauss, M. (1899). 'Essai sur la nature et la fonction du sacrifice', *Année sociolog.*, **2**, 29.

— (1904). 'Esquisse d'une théorie générale de la magie', *Année sociolog.*, **7**, 1.

Jevons, F. B. (1902). *An Introduction to the History of Religion*, 2nd ed., London. (1st ed., 1896.)

Joustra, M. (1902). 'Het leven, de zeden en gewoonten der Bataks', *Meded. ned. Zend.*, **46**, 385.

Jung, C. G. (1912). 'Wandlungen und Symbole der Libido', *Jb. psychoanal. psychopath. Forsch.*, **3**, 120 and **4**, 162.
(*Trans.: Psychology of the Unconscious*, London, 1919.)

— (1913). 'Versuch einer Darstellung der psychoanalytischen Theorie', *Jb. psychoanal. psychopath. Forsch.*, **5**, 307.
(*Trans.: The Theory of Psycho-Analysis*, New York, 1915.)

Junod, H. A. (1898). *Les Ba-Ronga*, Neuchâtel.

Kaempfer, E. (1727). *The History of Japan* (2 vols.), London.

Keane, A. H. (1899). *Man, Past and Present*, Cambridge.

Kleinpaul, R. (1898). *Die Lebendigen und die Toten in Volksglauben, Religion und Sage*, Leipzig.

Labbé, P. (1903). *Un bagne russe, l'île de Sakhaline*, Paris.

Lambert, Le Père (1900). *Mœurs et superstitions des Néo-Calédoniens*, Nouméa.

Lang, A. (1903). *Social Origins*, London. (Includes Atkinson, J. J., *Primal Law.*)

— (1905). *The Secret of the Totem*, London.

— (1910–11). 'Totemism', *Encyclopaedia Britannica*, 11th ed., **27**, 79.

— (1911). 'Lord Avebury on Marriage, Totemism, and Religion', *Folk-Lore*, **22**, 402.

Leslie, D. (1875). *Among the Zulus and Amatongas*, 2nd ed., Edinburgh.

Low, H. (1848). *Sarawak*, London.

Lozano, P. (1733). *Descripcion . . . del Gran Chaco*, Cordova.

Lubbock, J. (1870). *The Origin of Civilisation*, London.

McLennan, J. F. (1865). *Primitive Marriage*, Edinburgh. (Reprinted in same author's *Studies in Ancient History*, London, 1876.)

Totem and Taboo

McLennan, J. F. (1869–70). 'The Worship of Animals and Plants', *Fortnightly Rev.*, N.S. **6**, 407 and 562; N.S. **7**, 194. (Reprinted in same author's *Studies in Ancient History; Second Series*, London, 1896.)

Maori, A Pakeha [pseud. for Maning, F. E.] (1884). *Old New Zealand*, new ed., London.

Marett, R. R. (1900). 'Pre-Animistic Religion'. *Folk-Lore*, **11**, 162.

Marillier, L. (1898). 'La place du totémisme dans l'évolution religieuse', *Rev. Hist. Relig.*, **37**, 204.

Mariner, W. (1818). *An Account of the Natives of the Tonga Islands*, 2nd ed. (2 vols.), London. (1st ed., 1817.)

Max-Müller, F. (1897). *Contributions to the Science of Mythology* (2 vols.), London.

Morgan, L. H. (1877). *Ancient Society*, London.

Müller, S. (1857). *Reizen en Onderzoekingen in den Indischen Archipel*, Amsterdam.

Parkinson, R. (1907). *Dreissig Jahre in der Südsee*, Stuttgart.

Paulitschke, P. (1893–6). *Ethnographie Nordost-Afrikas* (2 vols.), Berlin.

Peckel, P. G. (1908). 'Die Verwandtschaftsnamen des mittleren Neumecklenburg', *Anthropos*, **3**, 456.

Pickler J., and Somló, F. (1900). *Der Ursprung des Totemismus*, Berlin.

Rank, O. (1907). *Der Künstler*, Vienna.
    (1912). *Das Inzestmotiv in Dichtung und Sage*, Vienna.
    (1913). 'Eine noch nicht beschriebene Form des Ödipus-Traumes', *Int. Z. Psychoanal.*, **1**, 151.

Reinach, S. (1905–12). *Cultes, mythes et religions* (4 vols.), Paris.

Reitler, R. (1913). 'Zur Augensymbolik', *Int. Z. Psychoanal.*, **1**, 159.

Ribbe, C. (1903). *Zwei Jahre unter den Kannibalen der Salomo-Inseln*, Dresden.

Rivers, W. H. R. (1909). 'Totemism in Polynesia and Melanesia', *J. R. anthrop. inst.*, **39**, 156.

Roth, H. Ling (1896). *The Natives of Sarawak and British North Borneo* (2 vols.), London.

Schreber, D. P. (1903). *Denkwürdigkeiten eines Nervenkranken*, Leipzig.

Silberer, H. (1909). 'Bericht über eine Methode, gewisse symbolische Halluzinations-Erscheinungen hervorzurufen und zu beobachten', *Jb. psychoanal. psychopath. Forsch.*, **1**, 513.

Smith, W. Robertson (1894). *Lectures on the Religion of the Semites*, new [2nd] ed., London. (1st ed., 1889.)

Bibliography

SPENCER, B., and GILLEN, F. J. (1899). *The Native Tribes of Central Australia*, London.

SPENCER, H. (1870). 'The Origin of Animal Worship', *Fortnightly Rev.*, N.S. **7**, 535.

—— (1893). *The Principles of Sociology*, 3rd ed., Vol. I, London.

STEKEL, W. (1911). 'Die Verpflichtung des Namens', *Z. Psychother. med. Psychol.*, **3**.

STORFER, A. J. (1911). *Zur Sonderstellung des Vatermordes*, Vienna.

TAYLOR, R. (1870). *Te Ika a Maui*, 2nd ed., London. (1st ed., 1855.)

TEIT, J. A. (1900). *The Thompson Indians of British Columbia* (*Jesup North Pacific Expedition*, Vol. I), New York.

THOMAS, N. W. (1910–11*a*). 'Magic', *Encyclopaedia Britannica*, 11th ed., **17**, 304.

—— (1910–11*b*). 'Taboo', *Encyclopaedia Britannica*, 11th ed., **26**, 337.

TYLOR, E. B. (1889). 'A Method of Investigating the Development of Institutions', *J. anthrop. Inst.*, **18**, 245.

—— (1891). *Primitive Culture*, 3rd ed. (2 vols.), London. (1st ed., 1871.)

WESTERMARCK, E. (1901). *The History of Human Marriage*, 3rd ed., London. (1st ed., 1891.)

—— (1906–8). *The Origin and Development of the Moral Ideas* (2 vols.), London.

WILKEN, G. A. (1884). 'Het animisme bij de volken van den Indischen Archipel', *Ind. Gids*, **6** (Part I), 925.

WULFF, M. [WOOLF, M.] (1912). 'Beiträge zur infantilen Sexualität', *Zbl. Psychoanal.*, **2**, 6.

WUNDT, W. (1906). *Mythus und Religion*, Teil II (*Völkerpsychologie*, Band II), Leipzig.

—— (1912). *Elemente der Völkerpsychologie*, Leipzig. (*Trans.: Elements of Folk Psychology*, New York and London, 1916.)

ZWEIFEL, J., and MOUSTIER, M. (1880). *Voyage aux sources du Niger*, Marseilles.

Index

168

Index

Index

Index

Prohibitions and underlying desires, 69, 70
Projection, 61-4, 92, 93
Psychical reality and sense of guilt, 159-61
Puberty ceremonies and avoidances, 10
Purification ceremonies, 20, 40

Ra, 79
Rain magic, 80, 81
Rank, O., 17, 130, 131
Razors, in a neurosis, 96
Regression, 17
Reinach, S., 78, 90, 101, 107, 113, 153, 155
Reincarnation theory of the Arunta, 114, 117
Reitler, R., 130
Religion: and father-complex, 145; origin of, 100, 142
Renunciation, 28, 34, 35
Repression, 30
Restrictions upon a victorious slayer, 36, 39, 40
Ribbe, C., 12
Richard III, 38
Rivers, W. H. R., 118
Roth, H. Ling, 81
Rulers: authority over nature, 43, 45, 48, 50; danger of contact with, 42-3, 48; godlike power of, 43-5; healing touch of, 42, 48; magic powers of, 41, 48; privileged, 47-8; responsibility of, 44-7; restrictions imposed on, 44-6; to be guarded, 41, 43-5, 48; to be guarded against, 41-3; unconscious hostility to, 49, 51

Sacrifice: 132-9, 147, 150, 151; and feasting, 134; animal, 133, 135-9, 151; by fire, 133; drink-offering, 134; human, 139, 151; in ancient Semitic religions, 132, 151, 152; theanthropic, 151, 152; vegetable, 133
Sacrificial meal, 134-9
Samoyeds, 54
Sancho Panza, 51
Sarawak, 37
Savage, Dr., 125
Savage Island, 47
Schelling, 76
Schopenhauer, 87
Schreber, D. P., 92
Scrofula, 42
Secondary revision and the construction of systems, 65, 95-6
Shark Point, 45
Shuswap, 53
Siberia, 54

Sierra Leone, 47, 49
Silberer, H., 150
Smith, W. Robertson, 132-9, 140, 142, 143, 147, 151, 152, 155
Social instincts, 72-4
Solomon Islands, 12
Somló, F., 110
Sophocles, 80
Sorcery and magic, 78
Soul: animals, 119; external, 116; primitive conception of, 76, 93, 94; transmigration of, 118
Spencer, B., 7, 114, 116, 117, 121
Spencer, H., 75, 77, 93, 110
Spirits: and the unconscious, 94; creation of, 93; doctrine of, 91; evil, 92
Stekel, W., 56
Storfer, A. J., 9
Sully, J., 90
Sumatra, 11
Superstition, 97-8
System-formation and secondary revision, 65, 95-6

Taboo: and conscience, 67, 68; and enemies, 36; and magic or demonic power, 21, 22, 24, 25; and obsessional neurosis, 26, 73; and penal systems, 20, 72; and symptomatic acts, 99; classification of, 19; meaning of, 18, 22, 66, 67; objects of, 19-20; on names, 54-7; on rulers, 41; on the dead, 51; on widows, 53; origin of, 31; punishment for violation of, 20, 21, 33, 71; sacred and unclean, 18, 25, 66, 67; sickness, 26; transmissibility of, 20, 21, 27, 28, 32, 34, 41, 72; Wundt's account of, 22-5
Talion, law of, 154
Tammuz, 152
Tasmania, 54
Ta-ta-thi, 5
Taylor, R., 28, 43, 58
Teit, J. A., 53
Temptation to imitate, 32-4, 61, 72
Thomas, N. W., 19, 83
Timmes, 49
Timor, 37, 39
Tinguiane, 54
Titans, 153-4
Toaripi, 39
Toda, 54
Tonga, 52
Totem: ancestor of the clan, 2, 104, 106, 108, 131; and blood-relationships, 3, 6; clan, 2, 103, 105; definition of, 2-3; eating of prohibited, 2, 104, 106; Frazer's account of, 103-6; individual,

171